CASE STUDIES IN TRANSPARENCY

REAL-WORLD WAYS
MARKETERS EDUCATE CONSUMERS

Maureen O. Larkin
Foreword by David Marlowe

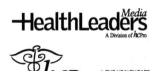

HealthLeaders *Media*
A Division of *hc*Pro

*hc*Pro | THE HEALTHCARE COMPLIANCE COMPANY

Case Studies in Transparency: Real-World Ways Marketers Educate Consumers is published by HCPro, Inc.

Copyright © 2008 HCPro, Inc.

All rights reserved. Printed in the United States of America.   5   4   3   2   1

ISBN: 978-1-60146-175-9

HCPro, Inc., provides information resources for the healthcare industry.

HCPro, Inc., is not affiliated in any way with The Joint Commission, which owns the JCAHO and Joint Commission trademarks.

Maureen O. Larkin, Author
Amy Anthony, Executive Editor
Matthew Cann, Group Publisher
Doug Ponte, Cover Designer
Janell Lukac, Layout Artist
Audrey Doyle, Copyeditor

Sada Preisch, Proofreader
Darren Kelly, Books Production Supervisor
Susan Darbyshire, Art Director
Claire Cloutier, Production Manager
Jean St. Pierre, Director of Operations

Advice given is general. Readers should consult professional counsel for specific legal, ethical, or clinical questions.

Arrangements can be made for quantity discounts. For more information, contact:

HCPro, Inc.
P.O. Box 1168
Marblehead, MA 01945
Telephone: 800/650-6787 or 781/639-1872
Fax: 781/639-2982
E-mail: *customerservice@hcpro.com*

HCPro, Inc., is the parent company of HealthLeaders Media.
Visit HCPro at its World Wide Web sites:
www.healthleadersmedia.com, www.hcpro.com, and *www.hcmarketplace.com*

Contents

Acknowledgments

I'd like to thank HealthLeaders Media for giving me the opportunity to write this book, and representatives from the healthcare organizations featured here who took time out of their schedules to talk to me about their organization's transparency journey. I'd also like to thank my husband, Mark, and my family and friends who were a great source of support through the writing and editing process.

About the author

Maureen O. Larkin is a contributing writer for *HealthLeaders* magazine and editor of the weekly e-newsletter *QualityLeaders*. Ms. Larkin is also editor of HealthLeaders Media's marketing strategy publication, *Healthcare Marketing Advisor*, and moderator for its "Marketing Service Lines" webcast series. She is a judge for the 2008 HealthLeaders Media Marketing Awards, and a member of the Society for Healthcare Strategy & Market Development (SHSMD).

Foreword

This is supposed to be an introduction to a well-written and timely book by Maureen Larkin on the state of transparency in the healthcare provider arena. In truth, it is probably more of an op-ed piece on my part. As you read this, please bear in mind that the issue of transparency is still very much in its introductory stages as I write this in the early part of 2008. I have little doubt that when I re-read the introduction some time in 2010 or 2011 I'll have a reaction somewhere along the lines of "boy, has that changed."

To start off with, what is transparency? To the best of my knowledge there is no official definition of transparency. But in a nutshell, transparency represents efforts by the healthcare system to provide key audiences (consumers, insurers, employers, etc.) with clear, useful, and comparative information that will help them make better and more informed decisions about where to go for health-care services.

What is driving this movement toward system-wide transparency? That subject is probably worth a book of its own but here are some key reasons from my perspective:

- The significant desire by healthcare providers to improve the services they are rendering to patients and all other key audiences—and to measure and prove that the improvements have indeed taken place.

- The drive by the purchasers of healthcare services—government, insurers, employers, and consumers—to make a more educated value decision when deciding whether to use Provider A or Provider B or Provider C.

- The desire by healthcare providers (and in particular hospitals and health systems) to differentiate themselves from competing organizations in a healthcare environment that often pushes provider entities into a commodity market position.

The issue of transparency falls into two distinct but related categories—information about quality and patient experience and then information about price. Taken together both information categories are essential for a true picture of value, but they often mean different strategies and challenges for providers.

One of the major challenges to the development and use of quality ratings is the fact that there is no single national or industry-wide standard for what makes up quality. In recent years there has been a growing level of consensus on some specific measures but these are hardly universal. As a result we have (to their credit) a number of hospitals putting forth their own quality measures through their Web sites and other outlets. We have state level outcomes results, the federal Hospital Compare data and numerous national rating services.

Many providers find it difficult to collect the information required to provide standardized quality information. Can we get what we need out of our information systems? Are the reports appropriately case mix adjusted? Do we have unusual outliers that skew the results unfairly? Is the sample large enough to be meaningful? And what is the cost of collecting, analyzing, and reporting all of this information?

A significant concern relative to quality information and ratings is whether the consumer audience understands the ratings. This is a fair concern. The information provided on Hospital Compare and other clinical quality rating outlets can be complex, even for clinicians trained to understand these issues. In spring 2008, as this book is going to press, there is a lot of hope that the new federal HCAHPS patient experience ratings will help this situation by providing a standardized measure in a language that is much closer to what consumers understand and can use in their decision making. The HCAHPS is meant to be the statistical equivalent of "talking over your fence to your neighbor." Only time will tell if this effort succeeds in creating a model that becomes the norm for consumers (and perhaps employers and insurers) to use in determining provider choices.

Another complicating factor is the level of competition that is going on among the various commercial rating services and among the organizations that receive the quality ratings. It is not unusual in some markets to see three or four different hospitals promoting their quality ratings from Rating Service A or Publication B. The jury is out on how effective this has been as a market differentiator for hospitals but it certainly is a key focal point for the marketing strategies of many provider organizations.

Finally, are consumers willing to use the available quality information, including the well known commercial rating services now on the market? While this issue is highly debated, it is my experience based on proprietary research done in 2007 and 2008 that consumers are currently not paying much attention to quality information and quality ratings.

- In quantitative studies, consumers who indicated that they have used a hospital in the past two years for clinical care were asked if they had utilized quality information or ratings from any governmental or commercial source (names of these sources were provided). Universally, the level indicating "yes" to this series of questions is less than 5%—and usually less than 3%.

- In qualitative studies (focus groups) consumers routinely express an interest in having understandable quality information but also express reservations about the nature of quality information and ratings systems current available to them. Key concerns that are routinely expressed include the understandability of quality information and the credibility of the information when it is known that some ratings organizations require hospitals to pay to get their results.

So if consumers have reservations about using existing quality information to determine which provider to use for healthcare services, should providers really bother (beyond what is needed to meet government or payer requirements)? In my opinion, the answer is an unqualified "yes" for the following reasons:

- We are only seeing the tip of the iceberg of the quality movement in healthcare. Virtually every other major purchase in our lives is supported by quality-related information, from buying a car to buying a house to taking a long overseas vacation. It is illogical and inconceivable that consumers won't eventually want some objective information to help them with what is perhaps the most expensive and important decision of their lives—where to get surgery or major medically-related treatment.

- Providing quality information—even if it has warts about your organization—is a way to engender consumer trust. Hospitals and the healthcare field as a whole have taken a fairly good black eye in recent years relative to consumer confidence and trust. Any transparency effort that will help to repair that breach is worth considering and implementing.

- While the percentage is small for those actively using quality information (including rating systems) to decide where to get health services, they (a) tend to be looking for more intense, higher-cost services and (b) tend to be better educated and better insured. Even attracting a small number of these individuals to a specialized clinical program can have a noticeable impact on the financial health of a provider organization.

- The internal effort involved in getting better quality rating scores or a top level rating or a "magnet" designation almost inevitably results in a better service being provided for patients—which after all is the true goal of the whole quality effort. In turn, winning such a rating or award is usually good for staff morale—who doesn't want to work for an organization that is recognized as being superior? And there are many studies that show that more satisfied employees result in more satisfied customers.

- Clearly payers (both governmental and commercial) are starting to take quality measures seriously. Pay for performance—including not paying for so-called "never" events—is here to stay.

As noted earlier, the other side of the transparency equation is price-related information. With some exceptions, price is very much the fifth and forgotten "P" of the healthcare provider marketing mix. But recent and ongoing changes in the American healthcare system have brought price more to the forefront. The number of consumers without health insurance continues to increase— and many of these consumers have jobs and steady incomes. The rising cost of healthcare is pressuring more and more employers to either offer high deductible plans and/or so-called consumer directed health plans. Either way, these plans place more of the up-front burden of costs on consumers. Related to this has been the growth of flexible spending plans that allow consumers to put aside pre-tax dollars for healthcare expenditures. It is not unusual to find many individuals in such plans sitting on significant dollars near the end of the year, facing a "use it or lose it" situation. Finally, there has also been a sea change in technology in the healthcare field that has allowed many more services to go "retail" and to be available on an elective (and paid out of pocket) basis for consumers.

One result of these changes has been a steady growth in price shopping by healthcare consumers. Ongoing proprietary research conducted in more than 15 markets across the country shows that between 8% and 20% of consumers report they've "price shopped" for healthcare. That level generally increases among younger (18–34) consumers, who are much more likely to either not have insurance or to have a high deductible plan. What this means is that in many markets, one household out of 10 is calling hospitals and healthcare providers during the course of the year to ask about the price of a diagnostic imaging test, a lab test, a physician office visit, an outpatient surgery procedure or some other type of care. And in all candor, most provider organizations are not well prepared to provide this type of information in a timely and effective manner.

This slow but steady increase in price shopping by consumers has not gone without notice. There have been many articles about this issue in both trade publications and major news outlets such as *The New York Times*, the *Wall Street Journal,* etc. There also has been an industry reaction to include some of the following:

- Mandates in some states for hospitals to post their prices on Web sites run by state agencies, hospitals associations, and other sources. In most cases, these prices represent hospital gross charges and thus are of limited use.

- Efforts by individual hospitals to provide actual out-of-pocket prices to inquiring consumers (including efforts profiled in this book by Maureen Larkin).

- A small cottage industry in firms offering to act as consumer brokers to negotiate prices in cases where there is a large out-of-pocket expenditure anticipated.

- Increasing competition from foreign providers, also called "medical tourism." Hospital providers in countries such as Thailand, Singapore, and India are actively promoting a variety of surgical services—and providing very specific prices (usually way below comparable prices in the United States). Moreover, some of these facilities are accredited by a division of The Joint Commission. At the time of this writing, some health plans in the United States have either contracted with these overseas providers or are in negotiations to do so—and are restructuring their health plan offerings to give enrollees incentives to fly 12–16 hours for surgical care.

As with quality information, developing and providing price-related information poses all kinds of challenges for providers. As a result, the movement has been slow to make this information readily and easily available. Two of the pioneers are profiled in the case studies presented in this book. Slowly, however, more providers are looking at price as a definitive strategic issue and not a byproduct of a charge master or bulk negotiations with a managed care plan. More are looking at proactive ways to provide consumers with useful and timely price information, at the very least for the services that are more likely to be "price shopped"—diagnostic imaging, lab services, physical therapy, outpatient surgery.

Transparency is a phenomenon that is here to stay for healthcare providers of all types. As a field, we will be faced with the challenge of providing quality and price information that is accurate, timely, and useful. We will also be faced with the challenge of what that information will mean to our market position, our marketing strategies, our operations, and our finances. This book contains eight cases studies of organizations that have taken proactive approaches to this very challenging issue. Maureen has done an excellent job of capturing the nature of their individual situations and how they approached quality and price transparency. I hope you find this information useful to you as you consider approaches and options for your organization.

David Marlowe has more than 28 years of healthcare planning, marketing, and business development experience as a hospital-based executive, consultant, and college level educator. He is a nationally recognized author and lecturer in the area of strategic healthcare marketing, including being the author of the recently published book, A Marketer's Guide to Measuring ROI: Tools to track the returns from healthcare marketing efforts. *Mr. Marlowe serves (in 2008) as president of the Society for Healthcare Strategy and Market Development of the American Hospital Association. He holds a master's of management degree in marketing and health and hospital services management from the J.L. Kellogg Graduate School of Management at Northwestern University.*

Griffin Hospital

Griffin Hospital is a 160-bed facility located in Derby, CT, with more than 1,300 employees. The hospital, which serves a six-town suburban area of southwest Connecticut, reported $310 million in gross revenue for fiscal year 2007 and is continually growing. You can find the hospital's Web site at www.griffinhealth.org.

Publicly reporting quality data isn't a new practice for Griffin Hospital. The effort is just a small part of the hospital's overall mission of patient-centered care, says William Powanda, vice president of the 160-bed facility.

"If you look at the overarching Griffin philosophy—empowering patients with information to allow them to make decisions—[providing quality data] is just a part of meeting that mission," Powanda says.

Griffin is a flagship hospital of Planetree, a not-for-profit organization started in 1978 by Angelica Thierot, an Argentinean woman fresh off an American hospital stay she described as "dehumanizing." After experiencing nurses who didn't look her in the eye and doctors who wouldn't share information about her care with her, Thierot envisioned hospitals that would "combine the best of spas with the best of hotels and the best of hospitals, to become a truly healing environment, where just being there is healing." [1]

Today, Griffin Hospital is the model for Thierot's vision. There's classical music playing in the parking lot, free valet parking, a baby grand piano in the lobby, private and semiprivate rooms, residential kitchens on every nursing unit for patient and family use, the smell of fresh baked goods in the hallways, daily massages, and many other amenities that truly make patients feel like they are staying at a fancy hotel instead of a hospital.

"Patients are less inclined to look at clinical information to rate a hospital than they are to the total experience, which they can understand and relate to," Powanda says. "The Griffin experience starts in the parking lot and ends in the parking lot. Everyone has to be a part of creating that personal experience."

Planetree comes to Griffin

The 1980s were particularly rough on Griffin Hospital. The hospital wasn't generating the profits it needed to invest in facility improvements, and its physical plant was the oldest in the state, Powanda says. Market share was falling fast, as was the hospital's ability to attract physicians, residents, and employees.

To make matters worse, a 1982 community perception survey asked, "If there was a hospital you would avoid, what hospital would it be?" Thirty-two percent of those who responded to the survey named Griffin as the hospital to avoid. Administrators knew the hospital would have to make major changes if it was to survive.

That's when Griffin decided to completely change its mission and philosophy to be more patient-centered. Griffin resolved to build a new facility that implemented the ideals of Planetree, but the road there wasn't easy. State regulators laughed at Griffin administrators when they saw plans for the new facility that included fish tanks, music lounges with pianos, open space, and resource centers.

"The obvious question was, 'Where did you get this idea?'" Powanda says. "When we told them it was part of the Planetree approach and it had been done in California . . . they said it would never fly in Connecticut."

But regulators changed their tune and allowed Griffin to go ahead with construction of the 100,000-square-foot inpatient care building, on one condition: "We had to build it at the same square-foot cost as other hospitals that were being built at that time," Powanda recalls. The result? "Some offices are smaller than our staff would like, but we used our space to create a totally different patient environment."

In 1992, Griffin Hospital officially became the first member of the new Planetree affiliate network, and in 1998, the not-for-profit Planetree, Inc., became part of Griffin's corporation. Today there are 95 Planetree hospitals in the United States and Europe, and Planetree's national headquarters is located on the Griffin campus.

Powanda says that today, interest in Planetree is at its highest point ever because of increasing pressure to improve the patient experience—likely prompted by public reporting of patient satisfaction scores nationally through the Hospital Consumer Assessment of Healthcare Providers and Systems (HCAHPS) survey.

Today, Griffin is a model hospital for Planetree, and its administrators often host officials from other hospitals who are curious to see the model that Griffin has in place. "Griffin is very different and you have to experience it. Until tour groups arrive here and hear the Griffin cultural transformation story and tour the facility, they don't appreciate it. We tell them all that this is not about building a facility; it truly is about changing the culture to put the patient first in all aspects," Powanda says.

A wealth of information

A patient who is admitted to Griffin Hospital is immediately given a packet of information about the hospital as well as his or her diagnosed condition. Within 48 hours of admission, the patient and his or her family members meet with the patient's primary care nurse and attending physician to talk about the diagnosis and the kind of care the patient can expect. For most diagnoses, patients receive information that describes in lay terms the tests, procedures, and care they will receive on a daily basis. And throughout their stay, patients are encouraged to look at their medical records, with the help of a staff member who can explain the information in lay terms.

Surprisingly, Powanda says, only about 45% of patients take advantage of the opportunity to review their medical records—a number that has held steady since Griffin began to offer the option. "I think it's an individual thing. I know if I were a patient, the last thing I would want to do is look at my medical records. My mentality would be 'Get me well quick and get me out of here,' but it depends on the patient's personal information needs," Powanda says. "It may just be one of those things where once it's made available, some of the mystery is gone."

Griffin also has a community resource library on-site that is open to the public, encouraging its patients to not only get involved in their healthcare, but also to really learn about their diagnosis and what treatment options are available. More than 15,000 people visit the resource library each year and it is considered such a health resource in the area that "the local public libraries don't even buy health materials; they just refer people to Griffin," Powanda says.

GIVING IT CONTEXT

Griffin uses the following to explain its infection rates and the measures it is taking to improve those rates on the Performance Indicator section of its Web site:

Healthcare-associated infections (HAIs) are a major public health problem in the United States and account for an estimated 2 million infections and 90,000 deaths. According to the Centers for Disease Control (CDC), a Healthcare Associated Infection (HAI) is defined as a localized or systemic condition resulting from an adverse reaction to the presence of an infectious agent(s) or its toxin(s) that a) occurs in a patient in a healthcare setting, (b) was not found to be present or incubating at the time of admission unless the infection was related to a previous admission to the same setting, and c) if the setting is a hospital, meets the criteria for a specific infection site as defined by the CDC.

In addition, Griffin outlines the ways it is working to combat hospital-acquired infections:

Hospitals, including Griffin Hospital, routinely practice infection control measures that are put in place to help reduce the risks of infection. Some of the control measures that we use are:

- Standard and Transmission-Based Precautions
- Use of antimicrobial dressings for specified central lines
- Total respiratory screening for all patients who undergo an operative procedure
- Interventions recommended by the Institute for Healthcare Improvement (IHI) such as:

- The "Ventilator Bundle" (practices to prevent ventilator-associated pneumonia such as elevation of the head of the bed at 30–45 degrees, daily sedation vacation and daily assessment of readiness to extubate, peptic ulcer disease prophylaxis, and deep vein thrombosis prophylaxis)

- Implementation of "components of care to reduce surgical site infections" (appropriate use of antibiotics, appropriate hair removal, and maintaining proper body temperature)

- The "Central Line Bundle" (handwashing, maximal barrier precautions, chlorhexidine skin cleansing, optimal catheter site selection, and daily review of line necessity to prevent central-line-associated blood stream infections)

- We conduct "targeted surveillance" which is data collected for selected infections. The infections that we have targeted are: a) Device associated infections: ventilator associated pneumonias (VAP), central line associated blood stream infections (BSI) in the critical care unit, and symptomatic urinary catheter associated urinary tract infections (UTIs) in the critical care unit (our numerator is based on the number of infections identified at each individual site and the denominator is based on the number of device days for each category); and b) Surgical site infections (SSIs) for knee arthroplasty, hip arthroplasty, colon surgery, abdominal hysterectomy, and vascular surgery (our numerator is based on the number of infections identified in each of the surgical categories and our denominator is based on the number of discharged patients who underwent a specific surgical procedure).

Posting quality data

The "transparent" healthcare that patients experience at Griffin continues with their online experience. Griffin began to publicly report its quality data around the time that it became a Planetree hospital, Powanda says, but its reporting significantly improved when the hospital launched a new Web site in 2000. The redesigned Web site included a Performance Indicator section, which Griffin has enhanced as more quality data has become available. "In 2008 there is an institutional goal to add as many as 75 new indicators," he says. All along, Griffin's philosophy has been to publish everything relevant to the consumer, Powanda says, regardless of the picture it paints for Griffin. "We underestimate the intelligence of the public to put information into perspective. We post everything—even information that may not put the hospital in a favorable light," he says. "And we don't suddenly pull something back if the rating drops."

Keeping less-than-ideal numbers online not only maintains Griffin's integrity in the eyes of consumers, but it also inspires the entire organization to work harder to increase scores in that particular indicator. Griffin not only posts the scores, but also explains their meaning and the efforts the organization is making to drive them higher.

Powanda says that communicating the information internally to employees and physicians is of equal importance. Monthly clinical performance data on Centers for Medicare & Medicaid Services (CMS) Core Measures and HCAHPS patient satisfaction ratings are distributed widely in a variety of forms emphasizing their importance to the organization and to creating an exceptional patient experience. Monthly HCAHPS ratings are posted in lounges on all nursing units. Sharing this information has resulted in improvement across the board, he says.

For Griffin, part of the Planetree philosophy is to not only give consumers data, but also give them reasons why the data is relevant to them. "The key is to . . . put [the data] in the context of what it means to [patients]," he says. "Otherwise, you could have people out there thinking our infection rates look really high, when in reality they're much lower than those at other hospitals."

Once the information was available online, Griffin's public relations department set to work, notifying the mainstream media and trade publications about the new information that was available. "Some of the reaction was, 'That's foolish, why are you doing that?' But we were ahead of the curve, as we typically are," Powanda says, noting that the sharing of patients' medical files brought a similar reaction when it was first adopted.

Surviving and thriving

Griffin hasn't just survived in this competitive marketplace, it has thrived, with continuing growth in admissions and outpatient visits and modest profitability eight of the past nine years. Griffin Vice President William Powanda attributes Griffin's success to its adoption of the Planetree patient-centered care model and its commitment to transparency.

Adhering to Planetree's methods has allowed Griffin to achieve industry-leading patient satisfaction scores, as well as dramatically improve clinical performance. Total Benchmark Solutions, Solucient/Thompson, HealthGrades, and most recently, the Premier Healthcare Alliance have recognized Griffin for its clinical excellence. What's more, Griffin received the Premier 2007 CareScience Select Practice National Quality Award for superior clinical outcomes and exceptional efficiency in patient care, putting it in the top 1% of the nation's 4,700 hospitals evaluated.

Competition

Powanda calls Griffin's service area "one of the most competitive in the Northeast." Located between three of the state's largest cities—Waterbury to the north, Bridgeport to the southwest, and New Haven to the south—Griffin is surrounded by seven hospitals within a 15-mile radius, six of them larger and with more capabilities. One of those is Yale–New Haven Medical Center, the state's largest hospital—which, because of its affiliation with the Yale University School of Medicine, has a longstanding reputation for excellence.

In its most recent community perception survey, Griffin ranked with Yale for the highest quality of care at hospitals in the region, Powanda says. The same survey also shows that more residents of southwest Connecticut are recognizing the benefits of Planetree. "A question in the survey asked the 400 people surveyed if they were familiar with Planetree," Powanda says. "Thirty-two percent said yes. More significant was the follow-up question, [which asked them whether they] could name a hospital that practiced the Planetree approach. Almost all of the thirty-two percent said Griffin. Clearly, they know Planetree, or know something about it. Planetree has become a brand that has clearly differentiated Griffin from other hospitals."

Griffin Hospital and HCAHPS

HCAHPS has issued preview reports covering patient experience surveys from discharges from the fourth quarter of 2006 through the second quarter of 2007. The reports from the nine-month period will be the basis for the first public reporting of results in March 2008. HCAHPS will move to a rolling 12-month reporting period in the next release of information.

Griffin Hospital's overall patient satisfaction in the preview report (percent giving the hospital a 9 or 10 rating) was 75% compared to the U.S. average of 63% and the Connecticut average of 62%. For the other HCAHPS groupings that will be publicly reported—Communication with Nurses, Cleanliness of Environment, Quietness of Environment, Responsiveness of Staff, Pain Management, and Communications About Medications—Griffin ranked 9% to 15% above (percent always satisfied) the Connecticut average.

"Griffin believes that a patient's HCAHPS overall rating is based on the total hospital experience and includes the many unique aspects of the Planetree patient-centered care model," says William Powanda, Griffin Hospital vice president. "It includes amenity services such as volunteers baking muffins and cookies in residential kitchens on patient units, massagelike rubs provided to patients, live entertainment including musicians and artists on nursing units, and a therapy dog visitation program. A fundamental belief at Griffin is that to provide an exceptional patient experience every employee is considered a caregiver," he says.

"We also recognize that programs, services, and information that were innovative and unique at Griffin five to 10 years ago are now the expectation for our patients. We are constantly raising the bar and looking for additional ways to enhance the patient experience," Powanda concludes.

Transparency and the turnaround

Adopting the Planetree philosophy brought the hospital that people in southwest Connecticut wanted to avoid to the top in terms of patient satisfaction. Powanda says the hospital routinely brings in patient satisfaction numbers in the high 90s and is continually working to keep it that way. The key, he says, is to always pay attention.

Griffin adopted the HCAHPS patient experience survey instrument as its sole patient satisfaction survey in 2005. It widely reports internally the ratings posted on the CMS Web site (*www.hospitalcompare.hhs.gov*), and includes the information on the Performance Indicators section of its own Web site. Later this year, Powanda says Griffin intends to add cost data to its Web site to further increase transparency for patients. Connecticut is a managed care–penetrated state, Powanda says, which makes it difficult for the hospital to give consumers an accurate picture of exactly what Griffin procedures will cost them. But he says Griffin administrators recognize the growth of high-deductible health plans in the region and the importance of having that information available to consumers.

"A lot of small companies in our service area have introduced high-deductible plans for their employees. Obviously, that is changing the interest level of employees in the cost of a procedure when they find out they have to pay for their colonoscopy out of their pocket because it would not be covered until they have met the deductible. In many cases, they are unaware of or don't understand the plan until they schedule the procedure," he says.

Consumers are already asking Griffin for cost information, and currently the hospital's business office is handling the calls, Powanda says. "We're seeing an increasing number of inquiries on a monthly basis. These calls used to be scattered a few years ago, but we get calls almost every day now."

The role of marketing

Griffin is different from other hospitals—and not just because of its mission and philosophy. There is no formal marketing department, Powanda says, and the institution relies on a data manager to collect and analyze the information the hospital needs to market its services. The rest is left to the communications and public affairs department, which develops and implements a marketing plan and maintains the Web site, including the Performance Indicator section.

Powanda says transparency isn't an effort that can be led strictly by marketers, though he feels that each institution is different. "I think it would be impossible for a marketing department to lead the charge and convince the CEO to post the information if it were contrary to the organization's ideas and philosophies," he says. "Every organization has its own culture—its own values and personality." Those values will determine whether a hospital is willing to share its quality, cost, and patient satisfaction data, Powanda says.

Conclusion

Of the 620 hospitals that have paid to tour the Griffin facility over the past several years, only about 20% have become Planetree hospitals. There are myriad reasons for this low number—from a misconception about the cost, the commitment, and the passion required to change the culture of an organization, to concern about achieving physician buy-in for an open medical record, patient care conferences for every patient, and patient empowerment. This is similar to the reasons a hospital doesn't adopt a practice of transparency or public reporting, Powanda says. "I think some of the things you hear are age-old myths and alibis, though I guess they may be the current perception of some hospital executives," he says.

Another common excuse is that the public isn't going to look at it, so why bother? "I don't know that all the public is going to look at it, but if it's up there, it shows that we have nothing to hide," Powanda says. He firmly believes that the wave of public interest will increase with HCAHPS. He describes HCAHPS as the next sea change for hospitals and an initiative that many hospitals wish would "go away." Although HCAHPS is voluntary, it is truly a form of mandatory public reporting because not participating will affect an organization's federal reimbursement rate. Public reporting of patient satisfaction ratings will prompt boards to demand improvement from nonperforming hospitals that will require an institutionwide response, Powanda says. "It's easy for the public, the media, health insurance companies, and legislators to understand, and it's going to resonate," he says.

Reference

1. "Under the spreading Planetree," Trustee, March 2007, p. 22–25.

Lessons learned

When asked to share the lessons Griffin Hospital learned through the quality reporting process, Powanda offers the following:

1. Develop a consensus vision that all constituencies support

2. Ensure that patient empowerment and transparency are organizational values

3. Consider everyone a caregiver

4. The environment demands being bold and innovative

5. Culture change requires passion, commitment, attention to detail, and continuing education and reinforcement

6. If this was easy, everyone would be doing it

Sentara Healthcare

Sentara Healthcare is a seven-hospital, 1,728-bed not-for-profit healthcare system located in southeastern Virginia and northeastern North Carolina. With more than 17,000 employees among its 100 different care sites and selection of health plans, the system reports a $2.5 billion yearly operating revenue. You can find Sentara's presentation of quality and cost data at www.sentara.com.

Customer opinion has heavily influenced Sentara Healthcare's presentation of quality data on its Web site, *www.sentara.com.* Over the past two years, Sentara has consulted with focus groups to determine exactly what consumers want from hospitals and how best to present that information to them.

Consumers were eager to tell the health system what they thought of different data presentations and tactics to make the information easier for them to understand. "We learned from consumers how they like to see information," says Lee Gwaltney, Sentara e-business manager, "so rather than [just] publish numbers and decimals, we publish charts and graphs that show a trend—not just what happened in one year or at one point in time."

Links to the quality and cost information are prominently displayed on the home page of Sentara.com, where users will also find a listing of quality indicators, along with descriptions of what each one means and why it is important. Even national awards—such as those from The Joint Commission and The Leapfrog Group—are explained for consumers, who are often confused by the claims made and rankings received by competing hospitals.

"I think a lot of time when there is publication of awards, [consumers] have a hard time distinguishing what is meaningful," says Cheri Hinshelwood, from Sentara's corporate communications office. By explaining how each award is determined and given, Hinshelwood says Sentara is helping consumers to see what is meaningful in what the health system is posting.

Sentara's site also makes sure to provide users with links to the agencies that collect data—such as Hospital Compare—to give consumers a place to verify the data. "We don't want to just trust that they're going to find Hospital Compare," says Deborah Roberson, RHIA, director of clinical effectiveness. "We want them to look at our information, but also [to] see that it comes from credible sources."

Engaging consumers

From the beginning, Sentara's staff knew the Web was the best way to engage the public in quality data, Gwaltney says. "The Web is the primary way that we're communicating this information and making it available. We've seen in our research that the Internet has been and continues to be an important place for consumers to get information."

When data was first posted in 2005, Sentara.com averaged 80,000 visits per month, Gwaltney says. Today, more than 111,000 visits are logged on Sentara's Web site on a monthly basis, showing the increased interest in the information Sentara provides. The Quality section of the site sees between 1,000 and 2,000 visits per month, he says. The health system has helped to drive interest to the quality information by placing direct links to the information right on its Web site's home page.

"We deliberately chose to put links on our home page and send the message that it was important," Gwaltney says. "We wanted to make it easily available for consumers, so they didn't have to look or search for it."

Finding the right way to engage consumers was important, says Gwaltney. All it took was asking focus group members questions and providing examples of ways that other hospitals present cost and quality information. "We went one step further than just asking what they wanted to see," he says. "We showed them examples of what things might look like—examples on the Web—and asked if they'd like a summary level of information or all the detail."

Focus groups

To best meet the transparency needs of consumers, Sentara used two focus groups when it was developing its Web content. It used the following criteria to select members of the two groups:

- Randomly recruited

- Ages 35 to 70

- Both males and females

- Must have been familiar with the Internet and used it to look up information during the previous three months

- Not employed by an advertising, research, healthcare, or Web design firm

Gwaltney says working with the focus group confirmed that those who use the Web are often scanners—when looking for information, they don't read every word, but rather scan the page they're looking at to find information. "Knowing this, we had to think about how we were presenting this information," he says.

Using a focus group also allowed Sentara to figure out what information consumers in its market segment wanted most, such as mortality and infection rates. The health system also learned about the research habits of patients, who asked to have more information about elective procedures such as maternity or gall bladder surgery, Roberson says.

Mortality explained

Sentara uses the following language on its Web site to provide background and context for consumers interested in the health system's posted mortality rates:

- When checking mortality for a hospital, the lower the number, the better. This applies to both mortality rates (% of mortality) and mortality ratios (actual rate compared to predicted rate).

- Look for a mortality ratio of less than 1.0.

- Only use mortality ratios that are "severity-adjusted," which minimizes differences among patients for a more accurate comparison between hospitals.

Gwaltney says focus group participants also expressed a desire to see more detailed data that Sentara hasn't yet been able to provide, such as data for more specific types of surgery, and data for specific surgeons. Although that information isn't available yet, he says the system is consistently looking for ways to give consumers more information and expects to offer more data in the coming years.

Prior to 2005, quality and patient safety data on the Sentara Web site was limited to select service lines, such as the Cardiac Outcomes Report. However, with the strategic focus to increase public transparency, Sentara expanded this information to initially include the evidence-based quality metrics that CMS and The Joint Commission were focusing on, such as heart failure and pneumonia care, with additional information continuing to be added based on feedback from consumers.

"It's the right thing to do to provide information to consumers," says Gary Yates, MD, chief medical officer. Sentara's entire community—staff, physicians, consumers, and members of health plans—should have this information, Yates says.

Sentara competes with a regional health system, an independent hospital, and a very large health system based in multiple states, Hinshelwood says. However, Sentara is the first in its market to publish quality and cost data. "Being a leader is clearly one of our initiatives. We knew this information wasn't available in the community, and we wanted to be the first to offer the information," says Roberson.

"I think being an innovator is an important part of what we do," Yates adds.

Transparency leadership

Sentara has two committees working to continually update and improve its presentation of quality and cost data. The steering committee, which is responsible for guiding the data presentation and making high-level decisions, is composed of the organization's:

- Chief medical officer

- Vice president of strategy, marketing, and corporate communications

- Chief financial officer

- Vice president of decision support/corporate planning and analysis

- Hospital champion for patient satisfaction

- Health plan vice president

In addition, a work group handles the tactical processes of making the data available to consumers. The following departments have representative membership on the work group:

- Marketing
- Strategy
- Clinical quality
- Corporate communications
- Finance
- Health plan

Sentara's leadership—including its board of trustees—was behind the quality initiative from the beginning. Roberson says that even physicians have given it their support. "We received no pushback from any of our constituents. In fact, we received full affirmation from our employees," she says.

Employees have embraced public reporting, and between hospitals, there's actually a bit of a friendly rivalry. Although Sentara has always had an environment that encourages patient safety and high quality, Yates says this rivalry has been the catalyst for improved quality and patient safety numbers. "As a health system, we've created an environment where we can learn from each other. There's a healthy internal competition that leads to better outcomes and patient care."

Encouraging patient involvement

Beyond the data available at Sentara.com, the hospital system has also developed sets of questions that patients should ask their physicians and other care providers. These questions change for specific procedures, but all have the same goal in mind: to involve patients in their own care. "Part of our education of consumers is encouraging them at every pass to take ownership of their experience," Gwaltney says. The "Questions to Ask Your Doctor" feature is among the top visited areas on the Sentara site.

Talk to your doctor

At Sentara.com, the health system uses every opportunity it can to encourage patients to communicate with their physicians about their healthcare. The following language is listed on the quality site, under "Mammography":

Mammography is an X-ray test of the breasts (mammary glands) that is used to diagnose breast cancer. The X-ray image is called a mammogram.

What you may not realize is that technology and expertise can vary significantly from one facility to another. Become familiar with the training, skill and capabilities of your imaging center and its procedures before you schedule your test.

Remember, you have a choice of health care resources and providers.

Here are some essential questions to ask that will help you make the best decision:

- How is your radiologist credentialed? Is he or she board certified by the American Board of Radiology?
- Exactly how much specialized training does your radiologist have? Does it include fellowship training in breast imaging?
- How long will it take your doctor to receive test results to help speed up your diagnosis and treatment?
- Look closely at the technology in use. Does your mammography center have computer-aided detection (CAD)?
- Talk to the staff before you schedule an appointment. Are they knowledgeable and able to answer your questions about the facility and the physicians reading your mammogram?
- How does your mammography center follow up a positive indication of cancer? What kind of technology is in use to assure you the best possible outcome?

Yates adds that he hears anecdotes from doctors that show patients are printing out these checklists and bringing them to office visits. Though no actual numbers are available, he believes the system is seeing the benefits of consumers who are more involved in their care. "A patient who is actively engaged and trying to understand [his or her] healthcare makes for a more active partnership," Yates says. "It's better for the health of that particular patient."

Marketing's role

Sentara's marketing department has been involved with the health system's transparency efforts from the start, holding a place at the table when the steering committee was created prior to the 2005 data release. The health system's marketers have been vital to the presentation of data.

"Part of our job [as marketers] is to effectively communicate our philosophy as a company—not just what we want them to know, but also what consumers need to know," Gwaltney says. The marketing department was heavily involved in the focus group work done early on, and from the beginning, it has been in charge of posting information online and developing related content.

"We're lucky to have marketing here because of its understanding of the Web and how it works," Yates says. When ideas are brought to the steering committee table, it's the marketing department that often translates these ideas into reality. "It is good to have someone in the room that understands the Web and its capabilities."

The Web posting efforts are just a small part of marketing's role, of course. "Our marketing team is really charged with the best mechanisms for reaching the population," Hinshelwood says. "They always have an appropriate tool that they can yank out of their toolbox to do this . . . they're the mechanism for getting information out into the community, and they partner with this team to get the information out there as well."

Adding cost information

Sentara added cost information to its online data presentation in December 2007. Feeling that the number of high-deductible health plans is growing in the market, Sentara officials decided it was time to offer consumers a way to figure out how much procedures will cost them. The link Defining the Costs of Healthcare offers consumers a place to request pricing information about a procedure they or a family member will be having in the future.

"Price and cost can be very complicated," says Gwaltney. Offering accurate pricing information has been a process that has taken time, but consumers looking for information are now directed to the hospital's finance department, which handles requests by phone. Patients are asked to have the following information available when calling:

- A copy of their current insurance card

- Their current deductible or copayment information

- The name of the facility where a doctor will perform the procedure

- The name of the surgeon and referring physician, and office telephone numbers

- Whether the procedure will be performed inpatient or outpatient

"We're monitoring feedback at this point. We've received a few—but limited—phone calls," says Gwaltney, adding that there's every indication that high-deductible plans are getting more prevalent in Sentara's service area. "We do know that consumer-driven health plans are going to grow," he says, noting that already some Virginians are enrolled in such plans. "We're trying to get ahead of it and provide information that's relevant to those folks as well."

Price isn't the ultimate factor in making healthcare decisions, Gwaltney says. Quality-of-care ratings and reports are just as essential for those evaluating their healthcare options. "We never think price should be an ultimate factor. Quality and information are essential in evaluating your healthcare partner," Yates adds.

The role of HCAHPS data

If consumers aren't yet engaged in the information available on Sentara's site, Gwaltney says he believes HCAHPS may change that. "I think people—as they take ownership of their health—are more readily looking for information about their health," he says. At press time, HCAHPS data had not yet been released, but once it becomes available, Sentara has plans to put the survey's data on its site.

The information that the HCAHPS survey gathers and the public reporting of it have the potential to really capture the attention of consumers, Gwaltney says. Customers are used to being able to log on to the Internet and find out how others rate a particular item or service. The number of people posting opinions and reading comments about auto mechanics, grocery stores, restaurants, and hair salons grows everyday, so why wouldn't consumers be interested in that information when it comes to their healthcare?

"I think [HCAHPS] is a place where people will be looking, because it hits home," Gwaltney says.

Conclusion

Although Sentara has no data that point to an increased number of patients coming to the health system since it started posting data in 2005, Gwaltney says that wasn't the health system's intention. "We like to think that providing information online does help navigate consumers to our system, but we don't have any way today to show direct correlation to information like that," he says.

Hinshelwood adds that a reputation survey done in 2006 may give an idea of what patients think of the health system sharing its quality data. "What we heard from consumers is that they trust us. They think what we're telling them is forthright and they trust the quality of this organization," she says.

In the near term, Gwaltney says the organization will again use focus groups when it revisits the Web site's features later this year in an effort to take it to the next level. "We're always asking questions, and we have a short survey on the site that some people have answered. We haven't really learned as much [from consumers] as we might have hoped, but we'll keep it up there as an easy way to ask questions of our consumers."

Sentara has had success communicating with its customers via its Web site, and Gwaltney says he has no doubt that is the best place to communicate with prospective patients as the healthcare landscape changes.

"One of the things that makes the Web most effective in delivering this information is that it's always changing," Gwaltney says. "I'm proud of our group and our efforts. We didn't post measures in 2005 and then take a year to update them. We update quarterly. This is the Web, and we want to make the information as current as we can. Keeping it accurate is the best way to educate the consumer."

Lessons learned

Throughout the quality reporting process, Gwaltney, Roberson, and Yates say Sentara learned the following:

1. The importance of establishing an internal infrastructure to oversee and guide the process. We sought multidisciplinary input across our organization, tapping relevant resources and expertise. Our steering committee provided the vision and commitment to support change and improvement. Operational support offered timely and accurate data and helped facilitate the internal improvement effort, while marketing provided a vehicle for effectively communicating via the Web and provide ongoing site maintenance.

2. Start small and engage the consumer early. Consumer focus groups provided valuable input into what data would be considered most relevant and meaningful. We also looked to consumers to offer formatting suggestions for better comprehension.

3. Set standards for the data. Our criteria included data being honest, accurate, and timely to support informed decisions. Where possible, we included comparative benchmarks to allow the consumer to put the data in perspective, and we expect data to enable consumers to become knowledgeable partners in their care.

4. Transparency is not just external—it must be integrated into the organizational culture. We believe supporting transparency is "the right thing to do" and will help us improve ourselves more rapidly. Data must be shared internally and frequently to leverage performance improvement.

5. Realize transparency is a journey, not an end. We put a great importance on continually engaging the consumer in the process and asking for feedback. Today, we are planning for the growth of information on our Web site, and we continue to design new ways to streamline data acquisition.

High Point Regional Health System

High Point Regional Health System has 400 licensed beds, and it serves the High Point, Winston-Salem, and Greensboro regions of North Carolina. The nonprofit hospital has 2,600 employees and reports annual gross revenue of approximately $500 million. You can find its Web site at www.highpointregional.com.

Over the past several years, High Point Regional Health System has learned a bit about what it means to be a quality healthcare provider. The hospital has been participating in the Malcolm Baldrige National Quality Award process, and it has discovered a lot about how it operates and what it can do better.

"You think you're doing extremely well . . . you look at this number and pat yourself on the back and say, 'What a great number,' but without context, we don't know if that number is any good," says Eric Fletcher, chief marketing officer. "Quality data has been such a tightly guarded secret that you never knew where you stood in comparison to other hospitals."

Fletcher says High Point's desire to compare itself to other hospitals made the organization realize that if hospital staff members were interested in how the organization stacked up among its competition, surely consumers would be as well. "Whether it's public shouldn't matter to us. The focus should be on what we're not doing well and how to make it better," Fletcher says.

Until it went through the Baldrige process, Fletcher says his organization hadn't made the commitment to compile and concisely present quality data. Located among many high-quality competitors, Fletcher says the area's consumers had an expectation that they would receive quality care regardless of which hospital they went to. Still, he recognized that consumers are increasingly interested in what kind of experience they'll have when choosing an institution. That's why in 2005, High Point launched its well-known and very popular patient blog site.

Patient blogs may not contain the latest procedure prices or quality indicator results, but they do enable consumers to learn more about what it's like to be a patient at High Point. "One of the things that we as marketers can do is help to improve the experience for our patients, and then, after you improve the experience, help communicate why that experience is superior to that [offered by] a competitor," Fletcher says.

Jenny and Sherrill's childbirth blog

The following is an excerpt from one of High Point Regional Health System's patient blogs, which have been sharing patient experiences with consumers since 2005.

The end–Part I

Stories, fortunately for some, unfortunately for others, have to come to an end.

Last Friday evening this pregnancy story ended with a 7 pound, 2 ounce, brown haired, blue eyed, and 20-inch long little girl named Olivia. But the power in a well told story is always in the way it concludes.

We arrived at the hospital Thursday evening . . . The hospital staff was ready for us considering that we had already done most of the paperwork when we went in for the "high leak" the week before. One of the nurses inserted a Cervidil into Jenny, Dr. Dorn visited, and the terrific nursing staff kept watch on her throughout the night, and I slept on the transformer chair/bed.

Friday morning, Dr. Dorn visited to see how things were going, the pitocin drip was started, and we settled in for a long day . . . the original birth plan was natural, with the option of "low dose narcotics," and an epidural only as a last resort. As noon came around, Jenny's cervix was not dilating as fast [as] we thought it should and the pain was starting to build, so she opted for "the drugs." An hour or so after taking them it was obvious that 1) she was high as a California redwood 2) they were only distracting her mind from the pain rather than alleviating it 3) they were not really doing the job. Under different circumstances I think that Jenny would have been reluctant about the epidural; however, it turned out to be the best thing that happened.

Seeing her lying there all hooked up to the machines, I think I really began to understand both sides of the birth argument. On the one hand, it was obvious that this was more of a medical procedure than anything nature intended. On the other hand, as one of our favorite nurses put it, "Having a root canal without anesthetic is natural too."

The nurse on the day shift really connected with Jenny, but her shift was over at 7 p.m. About 6:30, Jenny told her she wanted her to stay and help deliver Olivia. The nurse very politely told Jenny that while she was close (to giving birth), that she would be home helping her daughter move before ours was born. Although she was pretty sure that Olivia would not be coming in the next half an hour, she did agree to set up the room and help Jenny through some "practice" pushes. As we waited for a contraction, the nurse held Jenny's left leg and I her right. When the contraction came, she talked Jenny through. Two contractions later, I heard, "Oh look, there's the head!" Ten minutes later, we were waiting for Dr. Dorn and Jenny was being told to stop pushing until he got there. By the time he arrived, we were laughing, and she was ready to go. Olivia was born at 7:07 p.m., seven minutes after our nurse was supposed to leave. She was still there.

Allowing patients to give firsthand accounts of their hospital experiences is one way to communicate hospital excellence, Fletcher says. The increasing distrust of traditional marketing methods and the constant demand for information make blogs a great way to reach the public. "When we looked at those two things—transparency and distrust—it led us to think, let's focus more on the experience, and enlist the help of citizen marketers," Fletcher says.

"I think it's interesting to people because they want to see firsthand another's account of a service or experience that they're getting ready to face themselves," adds Aaron Wall, manager of public relations and marketing. "There's a certain amount of comfort in seeing that people have already gone through the experience that they themselves are about to go through."

Shopping for healthcare?

Wall thinks of the patient blogs as "consumer reports" of the services available at High Point. "I liken them to restaurant reviews. If I look at a restaurant review before I go, and it's written by someone who isn't an employee or [wasn't] compensated for their opinion in some way, it's more valuable to me," Wall says. "If it's a positive review, it makes me more likely to go there."

According to Fletcher, 20% of those who visit High Point's Web site access the patient blogs, which are categorized into three service lines: bariatric, maternity, and oncology. He adds that when the blogs were first posted in 2005, hits on the health system's site increased almost 25%, with bariatric patient blogs receiving the most traffic of the three service lines. "We can point to people who have decided to come here for bariatric surgery because of the blog," Fletcher says. Because of the size of the maternity and oncology service lines, he says it has been harder to track whether those blogs are bringing patients to these departments.

How it all started

High Point was one of the first hospital systems in the country to use patient blogs. "We try to stay well read on what's going on in public relations and marketing as an industry, instead of what's going on in PR and marketing in healthcare," Fletcher says. The idea came from a marketing journal about corporate blogs and what they could do. We just started thinking . . . in a hospital, you have wonderful relationships that you create with people. A blog would empower people to spread the word beyond their friends and families."

Perry, a 45-year-old man diagnosed with lymphoma, was the first patient to blog on High Point's site. Perry wrote about the tests and treatments he underwent in his effort to beat the cancer, and eventually used the blog to share his good news: In November 2005, he was given the "all clear" by his doctors. Since Perry's blogging experience, others have joined in, telling their stories of childbirth and bariatric surgery. At press time, eight High Point patients were actively blogging.

The blogs offer other benefits as well. One of the chief issues among prospective patients is how responsive a hospital or health system will be to their concerns, Fletcher says. The blog has been a vehicle to show that High Point's staff is highly attentive. If a patient blogs about something he didn't like about his hospital experience, High Point's staff will still post the entry, but staff members have the opportunity to respond—to explain what went wrong and what the health system is doing to make sure the problem won't occur again.

"It's a very public way to show people that we do address concerns and complaints, and we do it well and that people are satisfied," Fletcher says.

All of this work has not gone unnoticed. Years after the patient blogs debuted on High Point's Web site, reporters and researchers still call the public relations office to talk about the program and how it works. "When it first kicked off, we got articles and references in the *Wall Street Journal* and mentions in blogs across the United States," Wall says. "We even found blogs referencing what we were doing from as far away as Germany and France. We have a whole file folder of coverage." He adds that he's also talked with hospitals that are interested in setting up a patient blog program similar to High Point's.

The Internet dishes advice

At one time, research suggested that nearly 90% of American healthcare consumers reported they took their doctor's advice, Fletcher says. Today, research suggests that number is around 80%. "Twenty percent of consumers are willing to do some kind of research that may lead them to seek care at a hospital other than the one their doctor recommends," Fletcher says. "People have more information and are willing to question more than they ever have before."

Recognizing consumers' need for information, High Point has made its Web site a comprehensive resource for health information. Its Your Health section contains a prescription drug database, a symptom checker, information on complementary and alternative medicine, a medical test database, and access to Medline, the National Library of Medicine's database that provides links to more than 3 million articles.

Encouraging engagement

The introduction to High Point Regional Health System's Health Library includes a link to the organization's Medical Tests Database. Patients are encouraged to use the database to find out more about their health so that they can have educated conversations with their physicians.

> The Medical Tests database is designed to help you have a basic understanding of more than 200 common medical tests and procedures, to keep you better informed about your health and your care, and enhance communications with your current physician. Whether searching for information about a simple blood pressure test or a more complex Magnetic Resonance Imaging (MRI) test, this section will provide you with the facts you need, including a description, reasons why the test is performed, preparation, associated risks, side effects, and ways to understand the results.

Wall says High Point realizes that consumers can find such information in many places, but as a healthcare organization looking to meet the needs of consumers, he thinks it is valuable to consumers if they are able to find the information they're looking for at their hospital of choice.

"We want our community to be able to make informed healthcare decisions, and while they certainly can go elsewhere, we still want to make every effort to make that search for information as easy and efficient as possible," Wall says. "We have a corporate culture that aligns itself to the philosophy of 'Total Care' . . . it seemed only natural that we try and make our online presence follow that same philosophy."

High Point has also put electronic copies of its newsletters on the site so that interested parties can access them online—and can quickly find the subjects that interest them most. "It's formatted in such a way that users can choose what topics they're interested in," Wall says.

Coming soon: Data reporting

For the past three years, High Point has chosen to get on board the transparency bandwagon—but a bit differently than most hospitals. Instead of posting quality, cost, or patient satisfaction data, the hospital decided to focus on patient experience, because its marketing staff believed that experience is what matters most to patients. But as this book went to press, the system was actively planning to launch quality data on its Web site as well.

High Point's quality reporting will start out with the CMS Core Measures— heart failure, pneumonia, and surgical infections, among others. "[This] data is available to consumers now; it's just that it's not always that easy to find it on regulatory Web sites such as CMS. By putting it on our site, we're making it a little bit easier for people [to find]," Fletcher says.

High Point will also explain what each indicator means and why it is important to patients. "We are, in the briefest terms, trying to give the consumer information about what each indicator means and measures. We recognize that for a lot of our consumers looking at this data, some of the clinical terms aren't useful to them. We give them an idea of why this information is useful to them," says Wall.

For three years, High Point has been communicating its high patient satisfaction rates through its patient blogs, but once HCAHPS scores become available, the hospital plans to post actual rates and data. "HCAHPS should give a better apples-to-apples comparison" of High Point and its competitors, Fletcher says. "We'll report HCAHPS results and the results we get from [South Bend, IN–based survey administrator] Press Ganey."

Getting staff on board

High Point's physicians, nurses, and other medical staff members were in the process of reviewing the organization's quality data as this book was written. Fletcher says many were adjusting to the idea of this information appearing on the health system's Web site.

"Hospitals are very dependent on physicians and other healthcare providers to achieve high quality scores. Physicians are generally highly intelligent, very successful people who have never been told anything other than they're wonderful. When confronted with information that says the quality of care is lower in certain areas, it can be hard to accept," Fletcher says. "However, I have yet to find a physician who, when given good, reliable data that says there's room for improvement, has not made the effort to improve."

Sometimes, Fletcher says, the resistance is more about the need to understand where the data comes from. "Once they understand that the data is valid, they generally set to work to help us improve."

High Point's clinical staff leaders are hoping that public reporting of quality and patient satisfaction data will help the system's scores further improve, Fletcher says. "When you see a deficiency in a quality indicator, you can almost always trace it back to a process that isn't working the way that it should. If a data point shows us that we're not where we want to be or that we're less than we want to be, and we understand that it's a process problem and not a people problem, we'll improve much quicker," he says.

Will they pay attention?

Although High Point knows its patient blogs have captured the attention of consumers, Fletcher says he doesn't know what to expect when the system releases its quality and patient satisfaction data later this year.

"We haven't heard from our physicians that people are paying very much attention to the quality data that's already out there," Fletcher says. "I don't know if that's because it's presented in such a way that it gets lost, or people just don't understand it, or that they trust their doctors and their recommendations more than a Web site. So far, we haven't seen that the publicly reported data has made a huge difference in the way that people select their healthcare."

So, will it ever be a marketing tool for hospitals?

"It could be. When we're posting quality data, we're posting ours and the state and national averages, but I can see us one day posting ours and every other hospital in our area," Fletcher says.

Fletcher believes the government will continue to make federal reimbursement increasingly dependent on quality healthcare. In other words, hospitals will have to meet ever-increasing standards to get their full CMS reimbursement. A move such as this will make both hospitals and the public pay attention, he says.

Conclusion

Uncertain of the attention that consumers would pay to data reporting, High Point Regional Health System chose a different road to transparency when it began to use patient blogs in 2005. While reading and interacting with patient blog writers, consumers were able to connect with the organization through its patients, hearing about the experiences and quality care they had at the hospital.

By choosing a less traditional route, High Point Regional Health System successfully established a connection with consumers that brought new patients to the system and established High Point as a quality point of care in North Carolina. This quality reputation will be further enhanced later this year, when the system posts its quality and patient satisfaction data on its Web site—providing consumers with both personal stories and available data in one place.

Lessons learned

Following are some of the lessons High Point Regional Health System learned while using blogs to share the High Point experience with consumers:

1. Narrow your patient focus to specific experiences that occur over time. The best patient blogs are the ones whose experience becomes a journey.

2. Don't begin a consumer-based blog without knowing your organization and the service it provides. If you don't feel comfortable with the level of customer service your organization provides, it probably isn't a good idea for your consumers to openly journal about it on the World Wide Web.

3. Monitor but don't censor. We knew early on that no one would take us seriously if we approved or censored every entry posted. You have to be able to trust that your organization can make a positive difference in your customers' experiences, even if the initial feedback isn't positive.

4. Consistently seek new contributors. Because some people's journaling experience lasts longer than others, you need to be prepared with new bloggers to maintain consumers' interest in this highly interactive medium.

5. Read and listen to your customers' blogs. If you've taken the trouble to give your consumers the tools to give you feedback, certainly don't miss the opportunity to hear their free advice on how to better serve your public.

4

Lucile Packard Children's Hospital

Lucile Packard Children's Hospital, located in Palo Alto, CA, is affiliated with the Stanford University School of Medicine. The facility has 272 licensed beds and 2,498 employees. It reports an annual gross revenue of approximately $500 million. You can find its Web site at www.lpch.org.

Lucile Packard Children's Hospital is still new to the transparency game. It first started to post quality data online in January 2008, but did so after a long review process by its board, clinical staff, and consumer advisory boards.

"We spent a lot of time educating our board of directors about transparency and the role that it plays to improve quality and safety," says Paul Sharek, MD, MPH, medical director of quality management at Packard Children's. "Our board was surprisingly receptive . . . but they were particularly nervous about releasing data without information to guide consumers."

Guiding consumers meant that the board wanted the owners of the data being displayed to create context for every indicator presented—including an explanation of how the indicator was measured and what the hospital was doing to improve, Sharek says. "The board wanted to make sure that we were presenting data that was already being used to evaluate quality and safety throughout the organization . . . data that we were already continuously working to improve."

Packard Children's got similar feedback from its Family Advisory Council, a group of parents whose children at one time were patients at the hospital. Council members are specially trained to advocate for the hospital and work as partners with leadership in their efforts to improve quality and safety outcomes at the facility. During the transparency process, council members provided focus group feedback to the organization.

The council provided insight about the different levels of information that consumers are looking for, says Katherine Bryan-Jones, project manager for operations excellence. Some were looking for simple, uncomplicated information about the condition that they or a loved one was experiencing. Others wanted more detailed information that would allow them to do further research, but Packard Children's didn't want the data to overwhelm the parents who preferred less information. To provide this balance, the Packard Children's site shows the data graphically with simple explanations, but also provides links to additional information and details.

A hospitalwide effort

Thanks to a "trial run" of data reporting on the organization's intranet—available only to hospital employees—Packard Children's physicians and staff members were also able to give input regarding how the data was presented. Sharek says that 80% to 90% of the doctors he met with before the data went public "thought it was an excellent idea right away." The few who were more skeptical or concerned were converted after some adjustments were made to wording and to the information that provides context to data on the site, he says.

Packard Children's has had a philosophy of aggressively pursuing quality and patient safety for several years, so posting data online was the logical next step, Sharek says. "The initial reason for doing this was to really continue to drive improvements in our healthcare outcomes," Sharek says. Though it's too early to tell if the public nature of the data is driving higher-quality care at Packard Children's, Sharek says some anecdotal evidence suggests that hospital departments not only are keeping track of the data, but also are making efforts to improve it.

"The first call we received, after we went live with our transparency Web site, was from our own pediatric ICU. Due to a slight delay in our Web site launch, their data hadn't been updated to reflect their most recent outcomes," he says. "They saw the data and felt compelled to immediately address it. This suggests to me that the public release of our outcomes data is already showing signs that we're having the impact we were looking for."

Support from the top

The hospital's CEO, Christopher Dawes, was a critical supporter of the transparency initiative immediately, which helped to get the hospital's physicians on board, Sharek says. Dawes announced the hospital's intent to make data public during a meeting with approximately 150 of the hospital's clinical and administrative leaders.

"He promised the group that we would be transparent within the next couple of years," Sharek says. "It was a striking promise, particularly as the transparency concept was relatively new to healthcare at the time and my sense was that most people in the audience at the time saw this as more of a risk than it was worth."

But Dawes, who used to talk about printing the hospital's quality outcomes in the local newspaper long before healthcare transparency was promoted by quality and safety thought leaders, persisted. He invested a lot of time meeting with physicians and other hospital leaders to convince them that this was the right thing to do, Sharek says.

"He, our Vice President of Process Excellence Bradford Toussaint, and I presented our 'dog and pony show' to countless leadership committees," Sharek says. "Although the transparency concept remains a bit eccentric to some of our medical and administrative leaders, his efforts definitely helped."

Learning from others

While Sharek was busy convincing hospital leaders that publicly reporting data was a positive move for Packard Children's, Bryan-Jones was researching how other hospitals fared with their transparency initiatives. "I did a comprehensive Internet search to determine how many hospitals, particularly children's hospitals, had healthcare outcomes information available on the Internet. It was helpful to show our leadership which hospitals were already publicly reporting data, as well as what kind of data [was] represented," she says. Dartmouth-Hitchcock Medical Center in Lebanon, NH, and St. Louis Children's Hospital, and later, Beth Israel Deaconess in Boston, were three of the sites that helped shape the look and content of the Packard Children's site.

Bryan-Jones says this exercise showed her that if a consumer cannot easily find the information on a hospital's site, it might as well not even be there. "If I couldn't find quality data within a few clicks, I assumed it doesn't exist. Most consumers are not aware that this information is something they could be looking for, so it's important to have it right there on the main Web site. If not, and you have to really dig into a site to find the data, it defeats the purpose of the site and being 'transparent,'" she says.

To ensure that anyone visiting its Web site is aware of the availability of its data, Packard Children's has put a link to the Quality Data page directly on the home page.

Some good advice

Once they had drafted the content of the site, Bryan-Jones and Sharek turned to the hospital's Family Advisory Council. "We presented our initial draft of the site," Bryan-Jones says. "The parents provided excellent advice about how to explain complex data and ensure that our explanations were honest, yet 'family friendly.' Mortality ratio, for example, is a difficult indicator to explain, as no parent wants to hear that morbidity or mortality is a possible outcome. It was valuable to get parents' reactions to this type of information."

Once Bryan-Jones and her colleagues posted the Web site on the intranet and were preparing for the public launch, the Council again was asked for input. "They had a chance to walk through the Web site on their own and provide suggestions about the flow. It was interesting information to have from a consumer perspective," she says.

Although council members were mostly asked about the site's content and design, Bryan-Jones says they provided interesting information about how likely they were to use the information on the site.

"There were mixed reactions," she says. "There were some parents who are high-knowledge seekers who said this is exactly what they wanted, and that they actually wanted more data and explanations. These parents asked if we'd be putting more data up there and when. There were others who said they only wanted very basic information and that they might not have sought out this data without knowing it existed. But all of the parents pretty much agreed that if they were to go looking for that information, the Internet is where they would start."

Not your typical marketing tool

Sarah Staley, director of news and communications at Packard Children's, says the transparency process has not been considered "marketing," though her department did have a seat at the table when the organization was deciding how and why to post quality data. "It's not a direct-mail drop of an oversize postcard so that people will call up. This is not a sales tool," she says. "Our strategy is much more one of 'let's provide information, [and] enable and empower people to make educated decisions based on the most helpful information we can provide."

By giving consumers the information they're looking for, Staley says Packard Children's is making them feel as comfortable as possible with its physicians and facilities—something that is important to a family that is going through an emotional time. "We want parents to know that we get it. We want kids to forget that they're here to be poked and prodded. When families step into our hospital, we don't want them to think about data, infection, and all of those details," she says. "As well as we can give them a level of comfort and confidence [before they enter the hospital], the better off they will be from day one."

Staley says she's sure parents are using the Internet to research the healthcare facilities and physicians that will care for their children. She once volunteered for the local Ronald McDonald House—an organization that provides accommodations for patients and family members who travel long distances to receive care at specialty hospitals.

"So often, I would see parents in the computer lab just wanting to go online and see a picture of their child's caregiver," she says. "There's something about being able to see their faces. I'll always remember that, because it's really about finding the photo of what they're going to go through . . . that photo can show what kind of care they'll receive."

For many parents, it goes beyond the caregiver, and to the actual experiences that their children will have while receiving care. "When it comes to their children's health, they want to have as much information as possible. You're making decisions for that child. If it comes down to you making a decision for someone else's care, you want to make sure you're doing the right thing," she says.

Reputation goes a long way

Although Staley isn't ready to say that parents are already using the data available on Packard Children's Web site to make decisions about their children's care, she believes there is already interest in the safety of hospitals, particularly with the media reporting on medical errors and hospital-acquired infections. Quality care is important to all patients—not just their parents—and showing a track record of safe and happy patients can go a long way.

"I think it's important for institutions to be safe and continue to raise the bar of quality and make quality improvements," Staley says. A patient searching for a healthcare institution will want to choose one that is committed to care. Providing them with this information may not be a marketing strategy, but in some cases, it will help bring them in. "We're just going to continue adding additional data, and hopefully this information will empower patients to recommend Packard Children's to other families," she says.

Deciding what to post

Bryan-Jones says once the hospital decided which indicators it would post, the commitment was made to make the data available regardless of how high the hospital's scores were in that particular area. "We were clear from the beginning that this site was not intended to be a marketing site in the sense of only putting up the scores that made us look good," she says. "Rather, we released a cross section of data from our board of directors' quality and safety dashboard, and were committing to be transparent and honest with our results, even when we were not performing as well as we would like."

What we are doing to improve patient satisfaction

In addition to providing data and explanations of what the numbers mean, Lucile Packard Children's Hospital also uses its Web site to show that it is continually looking to improve quality and patient satisfaction. The information below is taken from the organization's Web site.

We are continually seeking improvements to move more patients from a "Good" to a "Very Good" rating. We are specifically working on areas we know are important to our patients:

- Improving patient satisfaction with how pain is managed and controlled, particularly with blood draws and IV starts
- Improving the discharge process by:
  - Better anticipating discharge times
  - Supporting patients and families through the discharge process
  - Ensuring comprehensive discharge teaching is completed so that families feel prepared to care for their child at home
  - Calling patients at home a few days after discharge to ensure the patient and family are doing well
- Investing in an electronic health record to reduce the repeat of information patients have to give
- Investing in facility improvements and hospital expansion to better serve the needs of our patients, families, and community

Showing the public that your scores aren't always perfect actually tends to build trust among consumers, Bryan-Jones says. She points to research conducted by Dartmouth-Hitchcock Medical Center, published in the October 2005 *Journal on Quality and Patient Safety*, that showed that providing honest and accurate data in and of itself was the key factor in engendering a positive reputation with consumers. Simply having the information available to consumers makes them trust the hospital more, and as Staley says, establishing trust among parents will make them more likely to bring their children to Packard Children's.

Putting it in context

When the board first gave its blessing to the hospital to publicly report some of its healthcare outcomes, it insisted that the Web site administrators make the information relevant and easy to understand by providing context for the data. "We provide basic information to explain what the data means," Sharek says. "Some of the healthcare outcomes data presently available on Internet Web sites is not presented with easily understood explanations."

At *www.lpch.org,* when a consumer clicks on "Re-admission Rate Within 31 Days", he or she is taken to a section that has a brief written explanation of what the indicator means—the number of patients readmitted to the hospital with the same diagnosis within a one-month period. The section explains that a lower number is preferable, and shows that the hospital's number, at 2.5%, is slightly lower than the 2.7% national average for children's hospitals.

"We've explained what it means for people who don't routinely interpret health data. Not all of the people who come to our hospital are familiar with this kind of information, so we wanted to keep the language as simple as possible," says Bryan-Jones. "The challenge is to explain [this] data in a family-friendly and simple way."

Understanding level of illness

Lucile Packard Children's Hospital sees some of the sickest patients in the nation, and therefore, outcomes are sometimes affected by the inability of doctors and nurses to treat a particular illness. To explain this to the general public, Packard Children's uses the following language on its Web site:

It is important to understand how patient populations differ between hospitals when looking at quality data. The severity of illness, or how sick patients are, at each hospital will have some impact on overall patient outcomes. Severity of illness is also called acuity. A standard measure to compare patients' severity of illness between hospitals is called the Case Mix Index (CMI).

Packard Children's Hospital has one of the highest CMIs in the country. We had the third highest CMI out of 76 children's hospitals in 2005–2006. In other words, Packard Children's Hospital cares for some of the sickest children in the country. We maintain very positive outcomes compared to other children's hospitals that see less sick children.

Marketing assisted in this effort, Staley says, making sure that the language was not only clear and concise, but also in line with the organization's usual communications style. "You never know what the spectrum of life is for the people that are viewing these pages," she says. "We have to think about how we address them as thoughtfully as possible . . . we see what the landscape is and what [consumers] are bringing to the table so that they can best do something with [this] data," Staley says.

When consumers log on to Packard Children's Quality Data section, they have the option of viewing a welcome video, on which hospital officials, including the CEO and the chief of staff, explain what the data means and why it is important for consumers. Shooting and editing the video was the job of the marketing department, and Staley says it is a preview of what is to come when the organization revamps its Web site later this year.

Video script

The Quality Data site for Packard Children's Hospital offers patients a short video that explains why the hospital chose to publicly report data and how patients can find it useful. The following is the script for the video:

Video: Christopher Dawes, president and CEO
Audio: Our goal at Lucile Packard Children's Hospital is to provide world-class care to children and expectant mothers.

Video: Outside shot of the hospital, patient/doctor shot
Audio: (Dawes voiceover) We want our patients, families, and surrounding community to have a true understanding of that level of care and our commitment to delivering it.

Video: Shot of the Quality Data site
Audio: (Dawes voiceover) One of the best ways for us to communicate this is by sharing our quality data with you.

Video: Thomas M. Krummel, MD; Susan B. Ford, surgeon-in-chief
Audio: Our quality data illustrates patients' and families' satisfaction with our services and the many different outcomes of the medical care we provide.

Video: Shots of the Web page
Audio: (Krummel voiceover) These Web pages define each quality measure, provide Packard Children's data, compare our results to any national standards that are available, and tell you what it all means. We also share what we're doing to improve our performance and the patient experience.

Video: Christy Sandborg, chief of staff
Audio: The honesty and accuracy of this data helps us evaluate and improve the way we care for our patients. The data reinforce accountability, reliability, and continuous quality improvement among our physicians and staff.

Video: Shots of the Web page
Audio: (Sandborg voiceover) We are continually working to improve in areas in which we perform highly, as well as those areas in which we are not leading the industry.

Video: Paul Sharek, MD, MPH, medical director of quality management and chief clinical patient safety officer; shots of *U.S. News & World Report*'s Best Hospitals issue
Audio: Some organizations have started to publish quality data on their Web sites, and we are proud to be one of the first children's hospitals in the United States to do so. We hope this trend will continue with other children's hospitals to ultimately improve care nationwide.

Video: Parent and child looking at a computer with a physician
Audio: (Sharek voiceover) We hope that you'll find this Web site's information useful and discuss it with your family and personal physician to make decisions about your child's birth or healthcare.

Video: Logo, screen with e-mail address: *qualityreports@lpch.org*
Audio: Music

Slow to catch on

For the first month of availability (through February 2008), Staley says the quality section of *www.lpch.org* has received approximately 1,000 hits. This relative lack of views could be due to a number of things, she says, including the lack of media attention it received when it was first released. "I don't think it's a sexy issue yet—having this information at your fingertips and using it to help guide healthcare decisions," Staley says. But she's not giving up. "We'll continue to communicate this as best we can, within the industry, or from time to time, if it makes sense, to do other communications with the media."

Sharek says the hospital's data has garnered the attention of other hospitals and insurance companies, which are excited about Packard Children's decision to post the information online. After only six weeks, Sharek says it's apparent what quality indicator holds the most interest—something that is very telling about what is important to patients. "Our most popular outcomes sites, to date, are related to patient satisfaction," he says.

Conclusion

Packard Children's representatives won't call the quality reporting process a marketing effort, but as a children's hospital, the institution must always consider the level of trust and confidence consumers have in the care that it offers. If the trust and confidence are supported and enriched, the hospital's market share will continue to increase.

Publishing quality and patient satisfaction data—along with simple, concise explanations about how the information was collected, what it means, and what the organization is doing to improve—only enhances the trust that the Packard Children's community has in its hospital. Consumer interest may have started out slow, but the hospital's location in the heart of Silicon Valley—with highly educated and sophisticated consumers—makes it almost certain that its Web site will soon be a popular place for consumers who want to learn more about the care their children will receive.

Lessons learned

Lucile Packard Children's Hospital learned the following lessons when preparing to launch its quality reporting initiative earlier this year:

1. Educate and then involve the board of directors as advocates

2. Spend the time to educate your executive, nursing, and physician leadership on why transparency is important

3. Engage consumers/patients in the development of your site to understand their needs

4. Show data both graphically and with a written explanation

5. Include a section on what the organization is doing to improve each indicator

6. Keep language simple and nonmedical

Alegent Health

Alegent Health is a nine-hospital health system with 1,832 licensed beds, located in greater Omaha, NE. The organization employs 1,300 physicians and 8,700 employees at more than 100 sites in greater Omaha. In fiscal year 2007, the system reported gross revenue of approximately $2 billion. You can find its Web site at www.alegenthealth.com.

When your CEO announces to 350 people that your hospital will be completely transparent by the end of the year, you'd better come up with a plan to fulfill this promise—and fast.

That's exactly what happened at Alegent Health in Omaha, NE. At a welcoming party for CEO Wayne Sensor in 2004, the leader told those in attendance that Alegent would be sharing quality data with the public by the end of 2005.

Rising to the challenge, Alegent Health's team responded. "In September 2005, we took out full-page ads and shared our quality scores, which we based on CMS Core Measures, and benchmarked ourselves against our competitors," says Amy Protexter, vice president of marketing and communications. "We averaged all their scores together and benchmarked what Alegent Health was doing."

That move started Alegent on a wild ride of sharing quality data that would position it as one of the leading health systems in the country when it comes to sharing data with consumers. Sensor speaks all over the country about the importance of sharing data with consumers, and earlier this year, the health system hosted a seminar called "Power to the Patient," which representatives of nine different hospitals attended.

"We very much believe in transparency," Protexter says. "That's the simplest way to say it. We've made a continual commitment to transparency and providing cost and quality data to consumers, but we're also very transparent with our medical staff and employees—it's a very pervasive philosophy."

Why transparency?

Sensor's announcement wasn't spontaneous, but something that he has been thinking about for a long time. "What I was really thinking was that there's a lot that is wrong with healthcare that is systemic in nature," Sensor says. "People are not very engaged in their health or healthcare decisions. There are a lot of reasons for this, but one of those reasons is because we've given them scant information to make informed decisions."

Hospitals and patients need to start thinking about healthcare as Americans do about other purchased services, he says. "When we think of the services that we buy as consumers . . . what other good or service do we buy that we don't know how good it is or how much it costs, but we're asked to buy it anyway?"

All of that is changing, Sensor says, and by making that announcement in 2004, he positioned his organization to be a leader in transparency. But the journey hasn't always been easy.

Resistance becomes routine

Before those full-page ads were released in fall 2005, Protexter says the system was careful to make all employees—physicians, nurses, and other caregivers— aware of the data and how it would be presented. "We wanted our physician partners to understand what was going to be seen," she says, "so we spent several months internally reporting and showing how the data would be reported."

"I would say that we painstakingly shared our intention—the rationale behind this—with our medical staff," Sensor adds. "We gave them the opportunity to offer suggestions and we shared our numbers so that our individual teams could test, retest, and begin to make changes."

Although most caregivers were quick to jump on the bandwagon, some offered resistance. When those full-page ads first appeared telling the public about Alegent Health's reporting effort, Sensor says some weren't happy with the CEO's transparency efforts. "The first time we published, it showed that our performance for heart failure for the largest tertiary hospital at Alegent Health was below [the] national average. I'll never forget one of the phone calls I got was from a cardiologist in our organization. He wanted to chat with me about what compelled me to pay for a full-page ad that steered consumers away from his practice and our organization," Sensor says. After hearing his concerns,

Sensor says he explained his reasoning behind the transparency efforts. "I don't know if I convinced him of our strategy, but I was very clear about who we are and what we stand for."

Today, physicians have welcomed the opportunity to help improve the health system, Protexter says, and they routinely monitor the data as it is updated. The result is a health system that has some of the best numbers in the country. "Our scores have literally soared to the point of perfection," Sensor says, "but it's not about bragging rights. It's about patients who walk through our door and receive the right care."

An easy read

Internally and externally, Alegent Health has come up with a system that makes the 30 indicators it reports user-friendly for consumers of all education and interest levels. The color-coded system shows how Alegent's scores stack up with national averages. "Green means we are where we should be, yellow means we're right below goal, and red means [we're] further below the goal," Protexter says, "so that everyone knows in what measures we need more focus."

Why quality scores matter

Alegent Health uses the following language on its Web site to explain to consumers why they should be aware of the quality statistics for their chosen healthcare provider:

Where you go for emergency care can save your life, or end it prematurely. According to a Johns Hopkins study of emergency departments, as many as 22,000 preventable deaths occur each year because emergency departments fail to follow proven treatment protocols for certain conditions.

In the study, 1,495 heart attack and 3,955 pneumonia cases at 544 emergency departments (ED) between 1998 and 2004 were reviewed. It showed that only "40% of eligible heart attack patients received recommended aspirin therapy, and only 17% received recommended beta blocker treatment. Among pneumonia patients, only 69% received recommended antibiotics, and 46% had blood oxygen levels assessed, as recommended by the American Thoracic Society."

Julius Pham, MD, an assistant professor of medicine in the Johns Hopkins departments of emergency medicine and anesthesiology and critical care medicine, said if this case sample were applied to all U.S. hospitals, he estimates "22,000 deaths a year could be prevented in the U.S., if ED caregivers followed practice standards." Alegent Health System quality scores for Heart Attacks and Pneumonia treatment protocols show our average is 99% or greater for both.

Alegent isn't hesitant to share those red scores, she says, because from the beginning, the plan was to share every score—good or bad. The organization started with 10 indicators tracked by CMS, and expanded it to "the Alegent 20" soon after. Sensor and Protexter both talk about expanding beyond the current 30. "We don't sanitize the data. What it is is how it shows up out there. The first time we published scores—in September 2005—we had scores that were below the regional average, and we shared them openly," Protexter says.

More than two years later, quality reporting is a part of Alegent Health's culture, and all staff members take responsibility for knowing the current sets of data and what's being done to improve. "We are at a 99%-plus score for every single indicator and every single diagnosis. Our board is monitoring quality at every meeting and we have process improvement methods underway. Transparency really helped us put focus and energy into improving our quality scores," she says. Protexter says a friendly competition has formed among the system's hospitals.

It didn't stop with quality

Happy with the results of the challenge he gave his staff in 2004, Sensor used a staff meeting to announce that Alegent would share not only quality data, but also cost data. He announced the My Cost program—a software platform created with MEDSEEK—which tells consumers how much a procedure will cost their insurance company, as well as how much will come out of their pocket. Sensor promised the program would be up and running by January 2007. It was.

"When you work through the tool, it tells you what your insurance company will pay and then what the patient's cost will be. It's relevant, meaningful information for them," Protexter says.

When developing the tool, Protexter says it was important for the data to really mean something to consumers. That's why Alegent went the extra mile to make sure payer information was included. "When we looked at others in the industry sharing chargemaster prices, we said, 'What does all this mean to anyone?' I think there was an internal 'aha!' that said, 'Why can't we build something that will tell consumers what their choices will cost them, or at least get them as close as possible?'"

Protexter adds that Alegent Health's team has been great at remembering to put themselves in consumers' shoes when delivering data—whether cost or quality—online. "What the consumer really wants to know is 'What is it going to cost me?' It's a simple concept, but one that the industry hasn't been able to get its arms around yet because of the complexity of our pricing system."

Why cost?

Cost is important information for consumers in greater Omaha, Protexter says, as several large employers in the region have consumer-driven health plans—including Alegent Health. In 2006, Alegent began to offer employees the option of either a health reimbursement account or a health savings account. In the first year alone, 79% of Alegent Health employees chose one of these options. Today, 92% of Alegent's employees are enrolled in a consumer-driven plan.

But Alegent Health isn't the only large employer in Omaha to offer such plans. Union Pacific and Mutual of Omaha both offer consumer-driven plans, and the number of people in Alegent's service area that are enrolled in them grows each year. Alegent Health decided it would be the leading provider in the market by offering consumers a place to find the information they needed to successfully manage their consumer-driven health plan.

Before My Cost was launched, consumers were often left to their own means to find cost information. "If you're not working in the industry, it's hard for consumers to fathom where to go to get this information," Protexter says.

The health system's billing department was handling price inquiry calls, but even the department's employees would have to do research to be able to provide consumers with correct information. "The nice thing about My Cost is that it's instant," Protexter says. "One of our competitors has a cost inquiry on its Web site, but they ask for 24 to 48 hours to call you back. With ours, you can find out how much something costs at one o'clock in the morning in your pajamas. My Cost puts control in patients' hands."

How to use My Cost

Alegent Health uses the following language to explain how its My Cost feature works at Alegent.com:

With any other major purchase in life, you know how much it will cost and what you're getting for your money. It shouldn't be any different with your healthcare. That's why Alegent Health puts the power of cost and quality at your fingertips. Simply visit Alegent.com and you can access objective quality reports and use My Cost, the first and only healthcare cost estimator of its kind in the world. They are the tools you need to make a more informed decision about your healthcare.

Before you start:
To receive the most accurate cost estimates, have the following items available:

- Copy of your current insurance card
- Current remaining plan deductible amount
- Current co-payment and/or co-insurance amounts

  1. Visit Alegent.com and click on the My Cost button.

  2. Enter your name and insurance or payment information.

If you have insurance:
Some insurance providers are directly linked to My Cost and will automatically enter your deductible, co-payment, and co-insurance amounts. If your insurance company is not directly linked, you will enter those amounts yourself. Simply follow the My Cost screens for instructions.

If you do not have insurance:
Answer a series of questions to see if you're eligible for financial assistance.

  3. Select the Alegent Health procedure you need.

Community reaction

In just its first year, Alegent Health saw more than 30,000 cost estimates created through the My Cost tool. Protexter says she expects that number will continue to grow as more businesses decide to go the consumer-driven healthcare route. "Though it was a little slow to catch on, our hits were strong on the tool for the first couple of months. We know our employees are using it, as well as the Union Pacific employees," she says.

The My Cost tool offers consumers a place to give input, and Protexter says that for the most part, they've received positive feedback. In fact, users thank Alegent Health for providing the information. "Before My Cost, there really was no easy way to get price information to help them make decisions," Protexter says.

Promotion and leadership

In a market where high-deductible plans are growing, you'd think Alegent's competitors would be right there in the thick of quality and cost reporting, but Protexter says Alegent Health was the first—and continues to be the only healthcare system reporting in the Omaha market.

"We heard last fall that one of our key competitors was working on quality reporting, but we haven't seen anything yet," she says, adding that because of the growing demand, Alegent expects its competitors will be scrambling to get information together for consumers. "I think they're all focused on what they should do and what they can do. We've been very proactive about it and are continually promoting our tools to consumers."

When quality reporting came online, Alegent used paid advertising to get the word out to consumers. "The quality story is difficult to tell," Protexter says. "In our industry, it's one of the things we all struggle with—what's relevant to consumers, and what kind of information we should share. Because we wanted to be able to tell the story in a way that we hoped people would understand, we decided to go the paid advertising route. We were prepared for and open to sharing the story with the media, but sometimes, on a story with complex data like that, relying on reporters to tell your story isn't the way to go."

When My Cost debuted, however, Alegent used the media to get the word out to consumers. "We got tremendous media coverage—local and national press," she says.

Are people paying attention?

Protexter says she knew that the My Cost tool would be used by those who have consumer-driven healthcare plans, but the growing number of Alegent Health employees choosing a consumer-driven plan leads her to believe that there are "natural shoppers" out there who are using the information available to them to determine where to seek healthcare—even if they don't have a consumer-directed plan. Those who have chosen these plans choose to be more involved in their healthcare, and the benefit of that engagement is showing itself.

"We've made tremendous progress in our effort to create a healthier work force. Hundreds of our employees have quit smoking. We have a very successful weight loss plan, and we see our employees better managing the more chronic health conditions," she says. "It's obvious that it is a good time to have consumers more connected to their healthcare. This was hugely lacking before My Cost and quality data were available to them."

That engagement is only the beginning. America as a whole is consumer-driven, and healthcare can't be far behind, she says. "Healthcare is one of the last market segments to not be touched by rampant consumerism. It's coming. There's more than enough information out there about what big-screen TV to buy . . . but soon [consumers] will realize that it's imperative for them to know how good the healthcare is that they're purchasing and how much it's going to cost."

Sensor says that in most markets, quality and cost data is not yet a marketing tool, but that time is not far off. "There are very few markets where people are going to choose based on that information, but more and more consumers will demand it," he says. "It's only a matter of time until we hit the tipping point, where consumers will make very informed decisions about who is best. If I think I'm a good provider and an efficient provider, then I should be comfortable with that."

Businesses get it

Sensor says transparency is gaining ground in one segment of every hospital's market: business. Beyond those that have decided to offer consumer-directed health plans, businesses are watching the transparency trend and are beginning to notice which hospitals are offering higher-quality care at a lower cost. "They're paying for half of the healthcare in this country," he says. "This audience gets it already. Our brethren in business and industry are very supportive of transparency and think it is a long time in coming."

Businesses believe that giving their employees information helps them make better, more effective decisions about their healthcare purchases—a move that could potentially benefit businesses in the long run. Sensor says marketers should take note of this because of the potential for partnerships between hospitals and business leaders to promote the availability of data and create better, more informed consumers.

The role of marketing

As Alegent Health prepared to release both sets of data, its marketers were charged with representing the consumer perspective. According to Protexter, they were asked how the data should be presented, how it would be benchmarked, and how people would use it to make decisions. "It's one thing to say, 'We scored a 95,' but what does that mean if you've got nothing to benchmark it against? On our site, we're committed to using consumer-friendly language and we wanted to build a site that would be relevant and helpful to consumers."

Though My Cost and quality information are no longer "new" news to the residents of Omaha, marketing is still working to get the word out to potential patients. Earlier this year, it launched a campaign featuring Sensor explaining all the tools Alegent offers a person to help manage his or her health. It also talked about ways that patients can be better healthcare consumers.

"If consumers aren't interested, it's our responsibility to help them. If you were to ask people from Omaha if they had seen scores from Alegent, most would say yes, they saw something. We've never given it to them before, but along with publishing the numbers, you have to help them constructively use it in their decision-making. It's our responsibility to help them get it," Sensor says.

Later this year, Alegent will launch another Web initiative aimed at helping patients become more involved in their healthcare. A patient portal that will enable patients to book appointments online, renew prescriptions, pay bills, and interact with others facing similar health conditions will launch. It is currently in its test phase, Protexter says, "but our vision for the patient portal is very broad."

Conclusion

The commitment to the empowered consumer is evident in Alegent Health's brand message: "This is your healthcare."

"Our brand, really, is all about empowering consumers to take charge of their health and their healthcare, but also about making sure we're designing a system that's easily accessible and approachable for them," Protexter says. "That includes providing tools like our quality and cost information so they can make good decisions."

That brand message has spread well beyond the hospitals' walls. Sensor has traveled all over the country, sharing his system's commitment to transparency and true belief in empowering patients. Even the staunchest critics haven't changed his message—and he's got an answer for every reason not to report this data publicly.

The reason he hears most often is that consumers just aren't interested, or don't get it. "I very passionately disagree with that. Whether you're a house-keeper or a white-collar executive, [you] buy goods and services every day," he says. All people are interested in making sure their money is spent in the best possible way—and they're more than capable of "getting it."

"I don't buy that argument for a second," Sensor concludes.

Lessons learned

Alegent Health learned the following lessons during its data reporting process:

1. Build the culture internally before you share information externally. Getting employees, management, and physicians on board is absolutely critical to your external success. Just as you design a thorough and thoughtful public relations or marketing plan, begin with just as robust a plan for internal communications.

2. Make the information meaningful and relevant to consumers. As you begin to share information, ensure that it will be useful to consumers in the format in which you intend to present it. Often, consumers cannot understand the way in which we share information within our hospitals or healthcare systems. The language we use is far too clinical and not consumer-friendly."

3. Whenever possible, provide benchmarks. Consumers appreciate that you will help them benchmark your data against other reliable sources. Think of *Consumer Reports*—which places a number of data points side by side—and you'll be on your way to creating tools that consumers can really use.

4. Share it all—the good, the bad, and the ugly. If you commit to transparency, you can't be selective if you also want to demonstrate integrity. As a side benefit, we found that when we reported scores below those of our competitors, it wasn't long [before] those scores were among the highest in our organization! Transparency motivates those lagging to improve.

5. Build on your success. Once you've tested the waters, learn from your efforts and continue to add measures to report on, additional procedures to share the cost of, and so on. Alegent Health is now tackling the addition of physician fees to our hospital-based and outpatient services, a frontier that many thought impossible to address. Yet our success along the way has helped [to] open those conversations with our physicians and challenged our team to "never say never" when it comes to getting consumers the information they need and want.

6

Geisinger Health System

Geisinger Health System, headquartered in Danville, PA, has three acute care hospitals, a drug and alcohol treatment center, 40 community practice sites, two research centers, a health plan, and 12,000 employees. Serving 41 counties in Pennsylvania, the hospital reports annual gross revenue of $1.9 billion. You can find the MyGeisinger portal at http://mygeisinger.org.

Like High Point Regional Health System, covered in Chapter 3, Geisinger has taken a different approach to the transparency trend. Although it reports quality data online, Susan Alcorn, chief communications officer, says the system does its best job of engaging consumers with its MyGeisinger health portal. Through *http://mygeisinger.org*, patients can communicate with their physicians; look at their health records; learn about illnesses, conditions, and treatments; make appointments; and renew prescriptions. "It's an entryway to our system. It allows patients to be more engaged in their healthcare," Alcorn says.

A site with many uses

As a user of MyGeisinger you can:

- Communicate with your physician by e-mail
- View lab and test results for yourself and members of your family
- View your online medical records
- Renew prescriptions
- Schedule and cancel appointments
- Read the most up-to-date information about health and fitness
- Get reminders from your doctor when it's time for yearly exams and immunizations
- Manage diabetes and other chronic conditions
- Check your account balance
- Pay your bill online

The portal does more than provide information, adds Patti Urosevich, director of national media. "They can interact with it and contact their healthcare providers. Some patients with chronic diseases are using [MyGeisinger] to report their conditions to their physicians daily," she says.

The site also allows patients to keep track of their vital statistics and shows them trend information. "You can monitor your blood pressure, cholesterol, and other diagnostic tests," explains Alcorn. "You can track progress and see if there are any trends."

The portal has been in place for four years, and in that time, almost 94,000 patients have used the site. It's a feature that is useful to patients of all ages, Urosevich says. The majority of the site's users are older than 35. In fact, 38% report being between 35 and 54 years old, and 24% are between 55 and 74. "Users vary in age," she says. "This isn't just a young person thing."

Physicians contribute to growth

When MyGeisinger first became available, it was simply a way for patients to find out test results online. Gradually, it has grown into a robust resource for patient information. Soon, Alcorn says, it will allow patients to have live, instant-message-like conversations with providers.

Physician involvement has been a key to the portal's growth, Urosevich says. Some physicians send secure e-mail to patients with chronic diseases to help them monitor their conditions. Other physicians share health-related articles with patients who may have an interest in a specific topic.

Most important, it was physicians—not marketing efforts—that helped to launch MyGeisinger back in 1998. When the portal first came online, Geisinger used billboards, radio, and posters in doctors' offices to gain consumer interest. "We tried traditional marketing tactics to get people enrolled, but it was slow going," Alcorn says. "Then we realized that patients were following their doctors' leads. So, we encouraged doctors and the support staff to take an interest in engaging patients in MyGeisinger. That approach has been very successful."

Most of Geisinger's physicians were on board right away, but Urosevich says there were some concerns about just how "in touch" patients would be. Some physicians feared that they would be inundated with e-mails, but that never happened, she says. Instead, most physicians found that the number of phone calls they received from patients decreased substantially, and they are easily able to triage e-mails to a nurse or other appropriate staff member.

Development of the patient portal was helped by the system's use of an electronic health record (EHR), Alcorn says. The hospitals and clinics have used an EHR since 1996. "In order to be a truly integrated group practice, we needed a means to ensure that care was consistent throughout the health system," she notes.

MyGeisinger's ability to connect with patients' health records paid off for one Geisinger patient, who was traveling in Maine when she was taken to the ER for dizziness, Urosevich says. With the help of the patient, the Maine hospital's emergency department team was able to pull up her health records and get a complete history of her care. "Access to the woman's EHR eliminated duplicate tests," Urosevich says.

The portal and transparency

For Alcorn, transparency is all about engaging patients in their healthcare: making them interested in the care they are receiving. "We believe that in order for patients to be as healthy as possible, and to get the best possible care, they need to be engaged in their own care. They need to be a partner.

They have to take care of their diet and exercise, and buy into the care plan. They have to have ownership of their own health," she says.

By putting the information at their fingertips, MyGeisinger allows them to do just that. At most health systems, it's a hassle for a patient to view his or her health record, but by becoming a registered member of the portal, patients can view their records as often as they wish—at any time of the day or night.

Alcorn says there are examples of this engagement throughout the portal, particularly with patients who have chosen to use it to monitor chronic diseases, such as diabetes and heart disease. "Chronic disease management—that's especially where it is valuable," she says. "For diabetic patients with fluctuating blood sugar levels, the patient portal keeps them connected. The office doesn't close."

Easy to use

From the beginning, Geisinger patients have found the portal very user-friendly. In fact, the ease of use has caused much satisfaction among patients, Urosevich says. "Moms love that they can download their children's health records for school recordkeeping, instead of having to travel to the doctor's office to get a copy," she says.

Alcorn adds that as a marketer, she sees many possibilities for spreading the health system's marketing messages with MyGeisinger. Though her department hasn't yet taken advantage of them, many of the system's physicians have. "If they want to remind you that you're 50 and it's time for you to have a colonoscopy, they can," she says. "Will we use it in the future for marketing? Yes, we will.

"Until the past few years, the way that people made decisions about their healthcare was that a doctor told them what to do, and I suspect that there are still people like that," she continues. "But there are more people searching around the Web to see what others are doing."

They're looking for a personal connection to their healthcare, Alcorn adds, and MyGeisinger, by providing easy access to providers and information, is giving them that. "People feel like they want to know about their hospital and their doctor. They know the information is out there. They feel like they deserve it, and they do deserve it," she says.

And the number of people looking for that information will only continue to grow. "Baby boomers are used to being online and are very savvy, and the younger generation has the expectation that you can get information 24 hours a day," she says. "My son doesn't wait to find what he needs. His age group does all of their surfing after 11 at night. They aren't waiting until the office opens at 9 a.m."

In addition to healthcare information, users of MyGeisinger also have access to their billing information, and Alcorn says the organization has spent a lot of time making its billing statements more user-friendly. Though the system hasn't yet promoted it in any way, users of MyGeisinger will later this year be able to access information about the costs of various procedures within the health system.

Conclusion

Geisinger's patient portal has been a success for the healthcare organization on many different levels. Spread out among 41 different counties in Pennsylvania, the portal has allowed effortless interaction between the system's community practice sites, research centers, and hospitals, giving Geisinger's care a "hometown" feel—no matter where care is being administered.

From a marketing perspective, the advantages of MyGeisinger are all about engagement and relationships. With the portal, a patient interacts with his or her physician as often as he or she wants—not just during a yearly physical. The tools offered by MyGeisinger encourage patients to think more about their own healthcare—whether it be monitoring their blood pressure monthly, logging their sugar levels daily, or keeping better track of family vaccination records. MyGeisinger makes healthcare less of a pain for consumers, making it more likely that they'll stay active and engaged.

Although the system acknowledges that offering patients cost, quality, and patient satisfaction data is important, building relationships is more important to the organization's guiding themes: quality, value, partnerships, and advocacy. And according to Alcorn and Urosevich, the MyGeisinger health portal is an example of the system's success in that regard.

Lessons learned

Geisinger offers the following lessons it learned while setting up its patient portal:

1. Engage physicians and the front office staff in enrolling patients.

2. Make navigation as simple as possible, and then test the site on an outside audience of varying ages. What seems clear and concise to an internal audience may be incredibly confusing to an outside one.

3. Include all stakeholders, including IT, in the planning process. No one person has all the answers.

4. Keep the site's messaging fresh.

5. Help the healthcare team consider new ways to use the portal, such as pushing information out to groups of patients.

Norton Healthcare

Norton Healthcare is the largest regional healthcare provider in Kentucky and southern Indiana, with four hospitals and a fifth expected to open in 2009. The full-service system has 1,857 licensed beds and approximately 9,700 employees. It reports yearly gross revenue of $3.2 billion. You can find its Web site at www.nortonhealthcare.com.

Norton Healthcare's brand message, "Expect more from a leader," promises the consumers of its market more—and since 2005 a commitment to true transparency and the online Norton Quality Report have allowed it to deliver just that.

Though it was not created as a marketing strategy, the quality report allows the system to be accountable to its community, improve patient care, and be a useful tool for consumers looking for resources to help make healthcare decisions.

Kentuckiana—the region comprising northern Kentucky and southern Indiana—is the health system's key service area. Its residents are well-informed, well-educated consumers who want to be involved in their care, and many are using the Norton Quality Report to make important choices.

"Female consumers in our service area are often the caretakers for their families," says Elizabeth Scott, associate vice president of marketing and e-business. "They are the ones making sure their children get their immunizations when they're due. They remind their husbands about upcoming appointments and screenings. They help an aging parent seek care when they need it, and they'll research the illness or condition of a family member to ensure their loved one is getting the right kind of treatment. For those consumers, quality reports will be yet another tool for them."

The Norton Quality Report is an interactive and educational report that displays the health system's performance on more than 500 nationally recognized indicators of clinical quality, patient safety, and patient satisfaction. "We believe that leadership should be transparent," says Scott. "If you say you're going to lead, present all of the information—the good and the not so good. It supports Norton Healthcare's position of integrity."

Norton's commitment to transparency has been driven by the healthcare system's top leaders from the beginning. President and CEO Steve Williams has been Norton Healthcare's leader since 1993 and with the system since 1977. He was the system's vice president of quality management from 1986 to 1988.

"Steve Williams' background and passion are quality," says Ben Yandell, PhD, CQE, associate vice president of clinical information analysis. "Quality has been Steve's focus his entire career. If you removed Steve's or the board's or our chief medical officer's commitment and encouragement from this equation, there would be no quality report."

An internal rollout

Public engagement, though important, was just a small part of Norton Health-care's transparency story. The story began internally, with an effort to educate physicians and the staff about the health system's level of care and how it could be improved.

When data was first shared with employees, Scott says the staff was told that the data would soon be available to the public and posted on the organiza-tion's Web site, *www.nortonhealthcare.com*. This was part of Norton Health-care's commitment to quality and transparency. "We knew we had to do this not only for our community, but also for ourselves," Scott says. "The focus wasn't on how the external community was going to respond, but how our Norton community—employees and physicians—would raise the bar."

Steven Hester, MD, MBA, vice president of medical affairs, says Norton's staff members had an "interesting" reaction to the news that the data would soon be released to the public: Every department wanted a piece of the action.

Norton made a commitment early on to only report indicators that were nationally measured. The health system said it would not create its own indi-cators, but instead would use those that were already standard practice. "Some departments didn't have numbers or metrics measured at the national level," Hester says. "They were asking, 'How come my department is not listed on the Web site?'"

Early interest in the data has continued as Norton has expanded its quality reporting process. "Our employed staff is engaged in our quality initiatives and they continue to be involved. There are metrics for each of them to work toward—they're meeting these outcomes and improving quality outcomes," Hester says.

Deciding what to include

Norton Healthcare's first commitment was that the system would report every indicator on each nationally endorsed list—there would be no "cherry-picking."

"If you start down the path of choosing which indicators to include, it's easy to convince yourself that the indicators you're flunking are also the ones that aren't important or that have definitional issues," Yandell says. "True transparency and selective reporting don't mix."

Norton's Quality Report principles

Norton's online Quality Report includes a list of guiding principles that were used when the site was developed. These principles are listed below:

- We do not decide what to make public based on how it makes us look.

- We give equal prominence to good and bad results.

- We do not choose which indicators to display. When we have a nationally endorsed list of indicators, we display every indicator on the list.

- We are not the indicator owner. We do not modify indicator definitions or inclusion/exclusion criteria in any way. We correct our internal data only for objective errors. We do not correct data submitted or billed externally unless we also resubmit or rebill the data.

- We display results even when we disagree with the indicator definition.

- We believe unused data never become valid. We recognize that we must display and make decisions based upon imperfect data, because until the data are used, no resources will be spent making the data valid.

Communicating this complex information is a challenge for any organization. Consumers, depending on their level of education and interest, would want varying degrees of information about clinical quality, whereas physicians want all the details. To solve this, Norton presented the information in a number of ways. Each indicator was color-coded for the easiest interpretation, supported by a numeric score that allowed the consumer to compare among Norton facilities, state and national statistics, and finally, a technical explanation of the details associated with each indicator. The different presentations of data allowed Norton to communicate to all interested parties—regardless of their level of education or interest.

With the color-coded approach, consumers could easily see in what areas Norton was scoring well, and those in which it needed to improve. If the system is scoring significantly above the national average, the quality indicator score is listed in green. If it's significantly below the national average, it's red. Scores near the national average are listed in a beige color.

"The data is complex. It can be difficult to get your arms around this, so we took a color-coded approach on our Web site," Scott says. "At any given time, you can look at a set of data and see how much red is showing for a group of quality indicators versus green."

Color charts are used to explain the numbers for each of the 500 indicators on Norton's site—including patient satisfaction, safe practices, and physician office care. Charts include a description of each indicator, the desired score, and scores for each of the four Norton hospitals.

An introduction briefly explains what each indicator means and how the health system is working to improve or maintain quality. If users want more information, they can click on each category listed, bringing up a window that further explains how the measure is determined.

Norton also made the commitment to continually update the data. By giving department leaders the ability to update the site as needed, Norton can ensure that consumers are viewing the most accurate, up-to-date information. "The online quality report provides great value, giving consumers information at their fingertips to use when making choices," Scott says.

A systemwide message

Once the public reporting plan was in place, Norton established what Scott calls an "elevator speech" that was to be used both internally and externally to describe what public reporting was and why the system chose to address transparency and a commitment to quality. It also named key members of its staff as "experts" who could field questions from the staff, the media, or the public about different sections of the reporting site.

"Questions about why, what, or how we were presenting quality data were directed to our chief medical officer. Questions about our methodology, statistics, or quality practices were addressed by our associate vice president of clinical information," Scott says. "To support the quality report from a marketing and public relations perspective, it was important that we knew who to direct questions to and that everyone understood the objective of the report."

When the report debuted, Norton informed the news media about what it was doing so that television stations, newspapers, and trade publications could help to spread the word that the data was now accessible to the public.

According to Scott, Norton Healthcare decided early on that it would not launch a formal marketing campaign around quality reporting, but instead would take a public relations approach. "This was not about marketing a service; it required supportive communication strategies," she says. "Public relations and communications were really the best ways for us to engage consumers."

Norton Healthcare's PR team set up meetings between the media and key players in the report's development to explain the initiative—what the information meant and why it was relevant to consumers. In addition, press packets were prepared and distributed. It was time well spent, Scott says, and adds, "We received very positive media attention."

"When people—the public, the media, and other hospitals—hear about our quality report for the first time, they're understandably skeptical," Yandell says. "They assume it's just self-promotion. Then they go to our Web site. They see indicators that are red. They see that we apply the word *worse* to ourselves. And they know they're not in Kansas anymore."

Most of the questions that Norton Healthcare receives about the site come from physicians or other health systems that are interested in setting up a quality reporting structure of their own. Rarely do calls come from the consumer at this point in the evolution of the report.

As for how the online quality report affects the direct choice a consumer might make, Scott says she's "not sure we're there yet, but we know that we're improving the patient experience by improving quality."

Hester agrees. "This is a first-round attempt. We're so very early in consumers understanding these metrics. As we work with the data and how it presents, we learn better ways to engage patients."

For now, Hester says, hospitals must continue to give consumers as much information as possible. "I think education is the key piece—as it is with so many things in our society. I can present lots of data, but unless I educate the user, it is of little value."

HCAHPS also has the potential to change patient interest. It will be different from other ratings systems because it has a standard list of questions, allowing hospitals to be compared "apples to apples."

Scott says Norton's continued effort to provide every patient with quality care will eventually bring consumer interest. "It won't be the sole deciding factor if they choose a Norton Healthcare facility or doctor, but it is going to become an increasingly important part of it," she says.

Quiet competition

Norton is the largest provider in a very competitive market, but almost three years after it first publicly reported quality data, local systems have yet to follow suit. "Pulling together quality data is really no small feat," Yandell says. "We're very fortunate to have the leadership in place to make that possible."

That's why—in an effort to allow consumers to compare apples to apples—Norton shares its data reporting approach with anyone who makes an inquiry.

For instance, both Kentucky and Indiana have state Web sites that share Norton's quality data, along with that of other hospitals and health systems in the states. Norton's information is also shared on the Web sites of other ratings organizations. Still, Hester says it's important for a hospital to present the information on its own Web site.

"We need to put this data out there because other organizations are going to put this information on the Web, too. Other organizations rate our health system, but they don't tell you how they do this . . . and sometimes they use older data," Hester says.

Norton's presentation of the data helps its customers understand what the data means and what the health system is doing to improve it. "By putting our information on our Web site, we can take control of our destiny. I really think that you have the opportunity to present the information in a way that helps consumers make a decision about their healthcare," says Hester.

Also, the continual process of updating and reporting data allows a hospital to act more quickly when data doesn't look as it should. Hester says that if data suddenly changes, the clinical staff can evaluate what's happening in that particular department and make needed changes to spur improvement.

Recognizing that smaller hospitals may not have the same resources as Norton to collect and report indicators, Scott says there are many other ways for hospitals to respond to the transparency trend. That response will depend on your hospital's culture. "It doesn't have to be a massive undertaking, just sincere, and a long-term commitment to transparency," she says. "Transparency can be as simple as having a town hall meeting with your CEO so that there's an open forum to answer questions."

In their own words

The following is Johanna's story, presented in the "Patient Stories" section of Norton Healthcare's Web site, *www.nortonhealthcare.com*:

I'm a woman on the move. After retiring from the railroad after 30 years of service, it's hard for me to slow down. Despite my physical activity and relatively good health, three years ago my doctor diagnosed me with high cholesterol. In addition to making some changes to my diet and encouraging further exercise, he recommended I start having regular heart screenings to help keep track of my heart health.

After a regular checkup with my doctor, I set up an appointment at the Norton Women's Heart Center. Although the center was a short drive from my home in Clarksville, IN, I wanted to go to a place that specialized in caring for women's hearts. I couldn't have made a better choice.

The nurses and staff at the Norton Women's Heart Center, especially Beth, are so kind and compassionate. I trust my heart to them, and they give me the reassurance and support I need to stay healthy; both physically and mentally.

With my heart in check, I can concentrate on enjoying my family and friends. I walk up to two miles a day, bike when the weather is nice, and work part-time at a thrift store in Clarksville. I enjoy staying active and visiting my son in Georgia. I've visited the center every year for my heart checkup, and don't plan to stop anytime soon.

She points to a section on Norton's Web site that tells patient stories. In fact, the health system encourages patients to tell their healthcare stories online, giving prospective patients an idea of what they can expect if they choose Norton for healthcare. "It's really about communication and being open with your community," Scott says.

Conclusion

Norton Healthcare has embraced the transparency movement and continues to grow its quality report. Like her hospital marketing colleagues, Scott believes that consumer interest in this data will increase—as more consumers realize that the information is available to them and take advantage of its availability online. Scott describes the target demographic of Norton's new hospital—set to open next year—as "progressive young families." These young families are part of the Internet generation, and are more likely than their parents to take advantage of information they find online.

Lessons learned

Norton Healthcare offers the following lessons that it learned while going transparent:

1. Remember that transparency has to be embraced not only by the leadership in your organization, but also by every employee. They are your greatest public relations team.

2. Plan all messaging several months prior to the launch of your transparency initiative. This includes consumer communications, employee communications, "elevator speeches," executive message points, presentation bullets, training materials, and comprehensive fact sheets that answer the what, when, why, and how of your initiative.

3. If your spokesperson is outside the department, train this person so that he or she is comfortable and on message when talking to the media about transparency's value.

4. Collaborate with colleagues outside of marketing and communications disciplines. Transparency rollouts are a group effort. Consider including legal, risk management, information systems, planning, or finance.

5. Set realistic deadlines and enlist the help of a project manager to coordinate the effort.

ProHealth Care

ProHealth Care, a two-hospital system located in the southeastern part of Wisconsin, has more than 550 licensed beds and 6,000 employees. The system, which prides itself on being the low-cost, high-quality provider in its market-place, reported $561 million in net revenue in 2007. You can find its Web site at www.prohealthcare.org.

When your health system is located in a competitive healthcare market with several noisy players, the best way to get the attention of healthcare consumers is to make your own noise about what differentiates you from the rest.

This was the strategy for ProHealth Care, which began publishing cost and quality data in 2002, says Clare O'Sheel, vice president of corporate communications and marketing. "One of the hallmarks of this hospital system is fiscal prudence. We've always done very well," O'Sheel says. "Because of that, we've been able to be the low-cost, high-quality provider in the marketplace."

ProHealth Care knew that it had a lot to offer the healthcare consumers of its region, but its leaders had to make sure that message was received by the community. That's why the system chose to not only make the information available online, but also to launch a marketing campaign to promote its availability.

Communicating quality internally

The majority of ProHealth Care's physicians, nurses, and caregivers were on board with cost and quality transparency from the beginning. "People were very proud about it. We did a big internal campaign about the value proposition and their role in helping to control cost and quality measures," O'Sheel says.

Employee involvement was a key part of the transparency process. Employees received messages about the value proposition in daily stand-up meetings, and their managers were sent weekly reports on employee efforts to reach their department's productivity goals. The bimonthly employee newsletter highlighted process improvement and cost-cutting efforts, as well as quality metrics. Managers were also expected to make the system's value proposition, "To provide the highest quality care for the most affordable cost," a part of their regular staff meetings.

A 2006 internal communications survey showed that 45% of the organization's employees could not only report that the value proposition was a strategy for the organization, but also recite it. The survey results showed that employees were "proud of it, and they backed it," O'Sheel says.

There were some unhappy physicians in the beginning, O'Sheel concedes, in that they questioned the health system's intention to advertise the publication of quality indicators that might not shine the best light on the hospital. However, today that discomfort has died down. "They understand it now," she says.

Throwing the first punch

In summer 2002, ProHealth Care published a brochure called "The High Cost of Healthcare." The brochure listed 12 common disease-related groupings for southeastern Wisconsin and, using Wisconsin Hospital Association data, compared the cost and quality of ProHealth Care's services to those of its competitors. The brochure showed that ProHealth Care's costs were well below one big-name competitor for both cardiac procedures and maternity.

The move was unprecedented, O'Sheel says, because at the time, the public wasn't thinking about cost and quality data when making healthcare decisions. They were, for the most part, seeking care at whatever hospital their doctor was affiliated with, or their managed care plan would pay for. Still, the hospital's revolutionary way of marketing itself captured national attention. "*NBC Nightly News* picked it up as a groundbreaking occurrence in 2002 in healthcare," O'Sheel says.

Promoting interest in cost and quality data

ProHealth Care uses the following language to encourage patients to take interest in the cost and quality data available on its Web site:

> At ProHealth Care, we take pride in the care we provide. We believe the reporting of hospital charges and quality measures are essential for employers and consumers making important healthcare decisions.
>
> Having charge and quality data at your fingertips enables you to make decisions with better information based on true value, and what the best value is for you. For us, having comparable charge and quality measures allows us to better judge our performance and improve our quality processes.

ProHealth Care's transparency journey didn't stop there, thanks to Ford Titus, the organization's "enlightened" CEO, who saw public reporting on the horizon, O'Sheel says. Over the next year, the organization set out to find more ways to present cost and quality information to consumers. Hospital leaders spent the year talking with hospital department managers and the medical executive teams to gather ideas about how to present the information. The health system also began to track how many consumer inquiries it received for cost or quality data, to determine the level of quality interest.

It turned out that consumers *were* calling for cost information, but the lack of a standardized reporting method was causing some misinformation to be given out, O'Sheel says. Leaders spent the next year devising a strategy for customer inquiries, deciding not only how the data should be presented, but also how the health system could keep it as up-to-date as possible. Once these methods were in place, all consumer inquiries were directed to the system's call center, staffed 24 hours per day by nurses.

Using this existing resource allowed ProHealth Care to deliver consistent messages, provide easy access, triage calls so as to direct inquiries to appropriate departments, track the nature of inquiries, and provide follow-up to consumers as needed. ProHealth Care tried this system on a trial basis for two months before announcing its availability to the public.

Quality enters the picture

After two years of marketing efforts that focused primarily on ProHealth Care's cost advantage, O'Sheel says the system wanted to make sure its record of providing quality care was also registering with consumers. That's why, in 2004, it started to publish quality report cards in three of its key service lines: oncology, cardiology, and women's services. The reports compared the care available at Waukesha Memorial and Oconomowoc Memorial hospitals to national benchmarks, based on data from the CMS and other repositories for quality data. The report cards also informed consumers about quality improvements happening at the hospitals and within the given departments.

The next logical place for ProHealth Care to present its cost and quality data was online, O'Sheel says, and in 2006 the information was posted on the Internet for the first time. The number of people visiting the system's Web sites (*www.prohealthcare.org*, *www.waukeshamemorial.org*, and *www.oconomowocmemorial.org*) and the rising popularity of the Internet made posting the information on the Web a "no-brainer," she says.

Since the Web content has been online, the number of inquiries to the call center has decreased dramatically. Most of the people looking for cost and quality information are turning to the Web, according to O'Sheel.

Deciding what to post

Before ProHealth Care's information hit the Web, a committee of representatives from different hospital departments was charged with deciding exactly what indicators would appear on the site. The committee was also charged with translating clinical language into a language that consumers of all educations and backgrounds would understand.

The committee decided that the indicators reported by CMS would be the chief indicators used to report quality on the site. O'Sheel says there was a lengthy discussion about what the system would do with an indicator if it cast the system in a bad light, but the final decision was to post all indicators, good or bad.

"The bottom-line rule was that we put it all out there. If you want to present the CMS heart measures, and one of them isn't good, you can't just take it out," she says.

HealthGrades

On its Web site, ProHealth Care explains how HealthGrades rankings work, and what a HealthGrades award means for the health system:

For the third year in a row, Waukesha Memorial Hospital's cardiac services are ranked best in the Milwaukee area, according to a 2007 study released by HealthGrades. Oconomowoc Memorial Hospital achieved a 5-star rating in heart attack management from HealthGrades, according to its 2007 study.

Because HealthGrades awards are relatively new, you may be wondering why HealthGrades is important and how the information they provide can help you make informed decisions about where to receive your hospital care.

About HealthGrades

HealthGrades, Inc. is the leading independent healthcare quality company, providing ratings, information, and advisory services to healthcare providers, employers, health plans, and insurance companies.

HealthGrades provides consumers access to information about the clinical quality and patient safety outcomes of healthcare providers and practitioners through its Web site and provides liability insurers, employers, and payers with critical information about healthcare quality and safety.

The analysis behind HealthGrades' awards is based on its Hospital Report Cards Methodology, which measures the care quality of nearly all of the nation's 5,000 hospitals in each of 28 procedures and diagnoses. HealthGrades analyzes the mortality and complication rates of millions of patient records contained in the most recent three years of Medicare data. HealthGrades then applies its risk-adjustment methodology so that hospitals receiving more difficult cases are compared on an equal footing with other hospitals.

The 2007 HealthGrades ratings for all hospitals nationwide are available, free of charge, on the Web at *www.healthgrades.com*. More than one million unique users and 125 major employers visit the HealthGrades Web site every month to access quality information about hospitals, nursing homes, and physicians.

HealthGrades also provides consumers and payers with detailed assessments of hospitals' patient safety outcomes, based on indicators developed by the U.S. Agency for Healthcare Research and Quality.

Starting with its first cost report in 2002, ProHealth Care used print advertising and direct mail to generate interest in the community and spread the word about the cost and quality information available. With each advertisement, O'Sheel says there was a flurry of activity at the information centers. "We heard a lot from the community. There were big spikes in call center and Web site hits whenever we would drop an ad or a direct mail piece."

One may ask why this two-hospital system in Wisconsin has been able to generate consumer interest while so many others have been struggling. O'Sheel says it may have to do with the area's demographics. Composed primarily of well-educated, well-insured individuals in a higher economic bracket, southeastern Wisconsin is full of people interested in learning all they can about their healthcare.

"Boomers are looking for quality information and cost information," she says. "With this cost- and quality-conscious group being a large part of our demographic, it really hits home for them."

How to use quality data

ProHealth Care provides visitors to its site with the following tips for navigating the quality information on its site:

- Familiarize yourself with the measures and how they can help improve the care that's delivered to patients.
- Review the methodology section of the Web sites. Are the results based on nationally recognized benchmarks and endorsed by organizations such as the National Quality Forum? Is the data audited?
- Be sure to look at the results over a period of time to get an accurate portrayal of organizational quality. One bad outcome in a quarter with relatively few procedures, for example, will greatly skew the results. Looking at three or four quarters provides a more accurate picture.

Another part of it may be the easy access to the information on the Wisconsin Hospital Association Web site. Although ProHealth Care's competitors haven't yet started to report quality and cost information online, the state hospital association has done so since 2005. The state site allows consumers to see quality, safety, and price information for hospitals around the state. "You can look up a specific procedure and it will tell you the cost and compare it to the state average. It's kind of neat," O'Sheel says.

With the state hospital association reporting quality and cost data, ProHealth Care could have just allowed the state agency to report its information, but by making the information available on your own Web site, O'Sheel says your hospital has the opportunity to give consumers more than just numbers. "They can come to our Web site and look up heart surgery, see what we offer, and the surgeons who work here," she says. Although the information on the state site is relevant, there are no "words and music with it. Just the facts," she says.

Will Wisconsin's interest spread?

O'Sheel acknowledges that not all markets are like ProHealth Care's—but she says she expects that's going to change. It's time for hospital marketers to get on board the transparency bandwagon, and to give consumers the information they need to make informed decisions. "People are clinically aware. They're trying to become educated about some medical issue that they're dealing with," she says. "Quality outcomes are important to most people, and if the cost information was available to you, why wouldn't you look it up?"

Baby boomers—the population of America that is on the receiving end of most of the healthcare in this country—are wise consumers, O'Sheel says. They'll shop for healthcare just as they do for other goods and services.

"We need to start looking at consumers as shoppers—that's what it's all about now and will be even more so in the future," she says. "I went to a conference last August, and it was all about making your hospital a destination hospital. There was a whole session about cost and quality information and another whole session on the amenities that you need to offer."

Hospitals that aren't paying attention to transparency are in danger of missing the next wave in healthcare, she says. "They're missing the boat. Change is happening. You can get on the boat and keep pace, or you'll get clobbered. The handwriting is on the wall . . . it will behoove you to allow patients to compare the costs of your hospital with others in the market. If you're not showing prices, people will believe that they can't afford your services."

Conclusion

Unlike many of the case studies presented in this book, ProHealth Care made transparency a marketing strategy from the start, and has seen great success. By touting its position as the cost and quality leader in southeastern Wisconsin, the health system has created better-informed consumers and increased its market share. Although O'Sheel says that there's no way to track the system's growth to its data reporting efforts, the system's market share has grown every year since 2002—the year it issued its first cost and quality report.

"We're still trying to track how many people are choosing us based on the information we have available," concludes O'Sheel. "We know that when we've done focus groups, people who were unaware that this information was available have said that yes, they would choose us based on this information."

Lessons learned

ProHealth Care says it learned the following lessons from its quality and cost reporting efforts:

1. If your CEO isn't the visionary for this, ensure his or her sponsorship.

2. Get everyone on the same page with a clear definition of purpose/philosophy.

3. Ensure accuracy by centralizing the response process.

4. Involve physicians, especially in determining the quality measures on which you will hang your hat.

5. Don't put this off. More and more of your data will be publicly reported. Position your good and bad news now.

The great disclosure debate

By Molly Rowe

Editor's note: The following story was originally published in the October 2007 edition of HealthLeaders *magazine. For more information visit* www.healthleadersmedia.com.

Reporting quality scores on certain core measures is common practice for hospitals, but senior leaders across the country are encountering mounting pressure from board members, regulators, competitors, and customers to take their data reporting a step further: full transparency. Hospital leaders and quality departments meet regularly to debate the whys and why nots of such disclosure, but few have pulled the trigger. With a small but growing number of hospitals opting to report quality data on their own Web sites, however, that could be changing.

Devil's in the debate

For hospitals still entrenched in the transparency decision process, the list of why nots is a long one: It will take too many resources. We already have more reports than we can handle. Consumers won't understand the data. The public relations and legal risks are too high. Senior leaders at Sinai Hospital of

Baltimore, for instance, spent more than a year debating before deciding they weren't yet ready to post quality scores on their Web site. "The more we discussed, the more we talked ourselves out of it," says Sinai Vice President Barbara Epke.

But transparency is a no-brainer for the handful of hospitals that have passed the debate stages and launched their own quality Web sites. Executives at such organizations argue that, when done right, a hospital-driven public reporting tool will actually improve customer understanding, reduce the redundancy of reports, and improve the efficiency of the quality department.

"Implementing a transparency initiative is easier than it's ever been. It's puzzling to me as to why people haven't gotten on the bandwagon," say Daniel Varga, MD, chief medical officer at SSM Healthcare–St. Louis. SSM's Web site currently provides data on patient safety, core measures; and hospital-acquired infections for its St. Louis–area hospitals, but the network plans to launch a more extensive quality site by the end of this year.

So why does one system choose to take the quality leap while others do not?

Board buy-in

In March 2005, Louisville, KY–based Norton Healthcare launched the Norton Quality Report, a section of the system's Web site that lists Norton's scores on more than 400 quality indicators. Norton's transparency push was driven by the board's belief in accountability. With the board's backing—and insistence—

Norton's quality stakeholders were free to focus their energies on delivery rather than debate.

That's when the real talking began. Norton's quality leaders educated the board and all internal audiences on what was happening and why. They invited local agencies outside of the hospital, including the local media, to be involved in the transparency process.

"We asked the press to be involved with us in the communication and education process, and we went through painstaking efforts for them to understand how the site actually works and how it was going to be an easy site to use. We had to convince them that this wasn't a marketing or positioning ploy," says Russell Cox, Norton's chief operating officer.

To publish or not to publish

The biggest decision delaying the move to full transparency for some hospitals, however, may be the question of which indicators to publish in the first place: How much data is enough? And can you post too much? This debate is what ultimately halted discussions at Sinai; senior leadership didn't want to post too few indicators, but they also feared that posting too many would overwhelm consumers.

Norton simplified the "what indicators matter" decision by creating a board-approved policy that says they will report any indicator that comes out as nationally recognized. Nobody debates, nobody votes—it is policy.

"This was not about us cherry-picking specific indicators that we thought would make us look good or promoting a specific service in any way. We were putting all of them out there," Cox says.

Norton's "all in" approach to transparency remains atypical. Most hospitals, like SSM, opt to begin with basic data—core measures, Press Ganey scores, infection rates—and build from there. Some only choose to publish measures that are reported already on other national or regional sites. But even that is a good start, experts say. "If we wait until we have the holy grail of indicators, we'll still be waiting two decades from now," Varga says.

Perhaps more important than what indicators a hospital actually posts is the explanation behind those indicators. Consumers don't always understand if a score should be high or low for a particular measure, Cox says, so it's important to provide clear and coherent explanations throughout the report—and internal staff should be able to understand and explain any data that is publicly available.

Linked in

Many hospitals not yet ready to publish their own quality scores—and hospitals still entrenched in the debate—use Plan B: Partner or link with an outside reporting organization.

"There are so many reporting requirements that hospitals have, it's all they can do to keep up with these requirements," says Beverly Miller, senior vice president for professional activities at the Maryland Hospital Association. Maryland is one of several states that have made reporting quality data a requirement of its hospitals. The data of all Maryland hospitals is posted through the Maryland Health Care Commission's Hospital Guide Web site. Area hospitals that don't host their own quality reporting Web site can link to the Maryland site instead.

Sites that are developed through a state partnership or links to other sites provide consumers with a comparative analysis of systems in the region, which can improve the usability of the information. "The advantage to posting your own data is that you get to tell your own story, but it's *all* your own story," says Alice Gosfield, a Philadelphia-based attorney and consultant who specializes in quality improvement.

Change is good

Regardless of how or when or where a health system chooses to go public with its quality data, senior leaders must be ready to react and make changes to improve outcomes. Clinicians want to be in the normal limits, Varga says, so if areas of the quality report are in the red, the hospital better be committed to making them green or risk losing clinician and physician support.

"The whole point of this undertaking is to speak to the quality of care provided in your organization," Gosfield says. "If you don't have the will to very explicitly improve the quality of care and then continue to keep raising the bar, you're having the conversation in the wrong place."

Thinking of going public? These three tips will simplify the process:

- **Set a date.** Hospitals should set a firm date by which they will publish their data. If you wait, you can let resistance build up to such a point that you'll never get through the process, Cox says.

- **Keep it simple.** When deciding what indicators to publish, don't invent anything, Varga says. Use indicators that have already been recognized and endorsed. Varga recommends using Centers for Medicare & Medicaid Services and Joint Commission core measures, as well as National Quality Forum and Agency for Healthcare Research and Quality measures, for a quick start.

- **Ensure data integrity.** Spend some time making sure you have valid data, and make sure your reporting is right. "If you go out and report indicators badly, it will take you years to regain credibility," Varga says.

Transparency: It's about the customers

by Maureen O. Larkin

Editor's note: The following story was originally published in the September 2007 edition of Healthcare Strategic Management, *a newsletter published by* HealthLeaders Media. *For more information on HealthLeaders Media, visit* www.healthleadersmedia.com.

Few days go by without another news report about one of the 50 states requiring its hospitals to post quality, cost, or patient satisfaction data online. Web sites now contain data about infection rates, mortality rates, and which doctors perform best when working on heart patients in California. Hospital executives are busily working to figure out a way to provide patients with the data they're demanding to make healthcare decisions.

Fueled by the rise in consumer-directed health plans, the transparency movement is one that's here to stay, says Carolyn Kent, a consultant with Cleverley and Associates, a consulting firm based in Columbus, OH, and author of the white paper *Marketing in Times of Price Transparency*.

Consumers have been forced to pay more attention to their healthcare, and now they're gaining interest in not only the cost and quality of your facility, but the total experience as well.

"Transparency speaks to the package of values that a consumer is looking for," Kent says. "Marketers have to constantly come back to understanding what consumers value and position themselves to deliver."

Responding to the transparency movement doesn't just mean posting pages of data on your site. It's about posting information that your patients want, in a way that they can understand.

What do they want?

Some hospitals are loading their Web sites with data about quality metrics, costs for various procedures, and patient satisfaction ratings from various organizations. Next spring, the federal government will release the first results of its own patient satisfaction data, the Hospital Consumer Assessment of Health Care Providers and Systems (HCAHPS), and hospital executives across the country are meeting to discuss their strategy for reporting these survey results.

But do cost, quality, and patient satisfaction data really affect how patients choose where to seek care? Healthcare marketing expert Anthony Cirillo of Huntersville, NC–based Fast Forward Consulting says no.

"Even with all the emphasis on transparency, I think it still comes down to where the physician recommends people go," Cirillo says. Most consumers don't care about—and don't understand—the cost and quality statistics offered by government and advocacy groups' Web sites, he says.

It's the total hospital experience that most interests consumers, Cirillo says. When considered individually, most people aren't interested in the data that tell them how often Hospital A's patients receive their medication on time or the average length of time it takes nurses to answer patient calls. Instead, consumers are interested in the total hospital experience—a collection of things that happen during their hospital stay and how they'll feel when their stay is complete.

Kent agrees. "A lot of Web sites I've seen simply repost information that is on the CMS Hospital Compare site, but try to put yourself in the shoes of Joe Consumer. If I have a heart attack and I get taken to your hospital, I know you'll give me aspirin, but what's the significance of that? For hospital marketers, it's a key question to answer. Help them understand what it means and make them understand that they will receive the highest quality care," she says. The trick, Cirillo says, is determining what information is most attractive to the consumers in your region. For a marketer, this should be easy to do, he adds.

"Create a culture of data collection so that people are telling you what to be transparent about," Cirillo says. If you live in an affluent community, cost may not be something your audience is looking for. If you're in a city with several well-known hospitals, patients may expect quality care from their hospitals and worry less about which hospital will provide them with the best care, Cirillo says.

Share patient experiences

High Point (NC) Regional Health System is one of those hospitals that has several high-quality competitors close by. "We have found in our region, from our own research, that quality is very much assumed," says Eric Fletcher, chief marketing officer for the 384-bed hospital. "The consumer has the advantage of having very high-quality providers, and the consumers assume that if they are going to a hospital here, that they are getting quality care."

Because of that consumer expectation, Fletcher says simply posting quality metrics on the hospital's Web site wouldn't do. That's why High Point Regional is using a different approach to responding to transparency: patient blogs. Since 2005, High Point has hosted patient blogs, encouraging those undergoing cancer treatment, giving birth, or having bariatric surgery to share their hospital experience.

"One of the things that we as marketers can do is help to improve the experience for our patients, and then, after you improve the experience, help communicate why that experience is superior to that of a competitor," Fletcher says. Allowing patients to give firsthand accounts of their hospital experiences is one way of doing so, Fletcher says. The increasing distrust of traditional marketing methods and the constant demand for information make blogs a great way to reach the public, he says.

"When we looked at those two things—transparency and distrust—it led us to think, let's focus more on the experience, and enlist the help of citizen marketers," Fletcher says.

Perry, a 45-year-old man diagnosed with lymphoma, was the first patient to blog on High Point's site. Perry wrote about the tests and treatments he underwent in his effort to beat the cancer, and eventually used the blog to share the good news in November 2005—he was given the all clear by his doctors. Since Perry's blogging experience, others have joined in, telling their stories of childbirth and bariatric surgery.

Offering patients a virtually unedited forum is risky, Fletcher says, but the hospital has only a couple of restrictions about what can be written on the site. High Point has some rules that prevent the violation of HIPAA laws, and writers are asked to avoid profanity, but otherwise, they are allowed to write whatever they wish.

"We've had situations where someone was blogging and had an experience that wasn't so great, and they said so," Fletcher says. "The patient had a long wait for a visit when they shouldn't have, and it gave us the opportunity to come onto that blog and explain the problem, apologize, and post a response." The key is how you respond to situations such as these, Fletcher says. By interacting with the patient's blog, executives were able to show the public not only that they care about what patients are experiencing at their hospital, but that they are committed to changing what's wrong with the experience. "And it humanizes us a bit," Fletcher says.

Showing that you can admit your hospital's weaknesses can indicate your hospital's commitment to giving patients the information they're looking for. "Openness reiterates the idea of transparency," says Kent. "It really adds a nice touch of humanity to the type of services that a hospital delivers."

Calculating patient cost

Dartmouth-Hitchcock Medical Center (DHMC) in Lebanon, NH, is one of those hospitals that has loaded its Web site with pages of quality, cost, and patient satisfaction data. But DHMC's site has been designed in a way that gives patients the tools to determine what the data mean for them. One of these tools is an out-of-pocket cost estimator (*www.dhmc.org/goto/charges*). Through a series of questions, the estimator helps patients figure out how much different procedures will cost them, factoring in their health insurance or lack thereof.

"It gives individuals some grasp of the cost of healthcare and a picture of the whole expenditure of resources around delivering a service that they very much need," says Melanie Mastanduno, BSN, MPH, director of quality measurement. She says DHMC wants patients to be able to factor cost into their healthcare decision process instead of making it their last priority.

"When there's an elective procedure in which they actually may make a plan for timing, this is very helpful information," says Mastanduno.

DHMC also provides information about the hospital's financial assistance program and allows the consumer to determine whether they qualify right on the Web site.

"We want individuals to not think of price as a barrier, but [as] one additional component to the decision," she says.

DHMC has been offering this information to its patients for the past 15 years through its call center but went online with costs in February 2005. Before showing costs, DHMC started with quality information, including procedures such as bone marrow transplants: survival rates, satisfaction data, how many patients experienced complications, and the typical length of stay, Mastanduno says. It immediately got a positive response.

"It's what they really wanted to know," she says. Seeing the data answered questions patients had and provided them with information that allowed them to plan for their procedure. "And our providers say it's helpful because patients come to them and already have questions in mind."

Since then, DHMC has consistently added new information to its site and is getting approximately 10,000 hits per month, says Mastanduno.

"There's no question that this trend is all over the national media," she says. "So consumers are much more aware."

So how did DHMC determine that the out-of-pocket cost estimator was a service worth providing for patients? It asked them. Before any data are included on the Web site, DHMC gathers employee and patient focus groups to discuss new content.

"Quickly, there was an excitement factor about how they could interact with the tool," she says. For those with high-deductible health plans, the calculator allowed them to more quickly understand the costs they would be responsible for.

And the Web traffic data that DHMC receives show that the cost estimator is being used heavily by consumers, Mastanduno says.

"We are finding about 25% of the hits for some of the different Web pages—mainly the cancer pages—are happening between 11 p.m. and 7 a.m.," she says. "Those are not our competitors surfing the Web in the middle of the night. Those are real patients looking for information on the conditions that affect them."

Like High Point Regional, Mastanduno says DHMC is committed to showing quality results regardless of what the scores say. For example, only 62% of patients receiving surgery for a herniated disc report that the treatment has given the pain relief they expected. This statistic is posted on DHMC's site, and Mastanduno says she often gets e-mails from consumers asking about the numbers. Having that result online is a perfect example of how committed DHMC is to transparency, she says.

"When people see numbers that aren't in the 90s or at 100, they actually trust us more," she says. "If we're going to be transparent, we're hoping to show a fair, balanced set of indicators. If we need improvement, we're going to say we are working on it."

Where do you begin?

Despite data that show patients aren't clamoring for cost, quality, and patient satisfaction numbers just yet, marketers say the time to develop your hospital's strategy is now.

"It's coming, so if we don't jump in front of it and lead it, it will be dictated to us . . . by the government or coalitions or whatever it may be," says Fletcher. "That's a situation none of us wants." Taking the lead in this process will only help your hospital in the long run, he says.

If your hospital hasn't yet developed a strategy to deal with the transparency trend, Mastanduno says the first step is to get support from the hospital's leadership.

"[Its] patients and [its] prospective patients have the right to know this information as part of their healthcare decision-making process," she says. "Our executive leadership said that from the beginning. If the opportunity is out there to have this kind of dialogue with your patients and your public, your leadership needs to stand up and say, 'We're going to take part in that dialogue.'"

The second step, of course, is knowing what data to provide for patients. Beyond advertising, this is the type of marketing that requires real, important communications with customers, she says.

"It's about having communications with our patients and our prospective patients," Mastanduno says. "It's a partnership."

Riding the wave

Here are some other examples of ways that hospitals are responding to the transparency trend:

- Cleveland Clinic, which was visited by more than 3 million patients in 2006, hired a chief experience officer in June to oversee all aspects of the patient experience. According to a Cleveland Clinic release, the chief experience officer will "advance Cleveland Clinic's patient-first initiative by creating a culture that addresses the emotional and physical experience for the patient, restore empathy as a core value, and recognize the central role that employees play in delivering an exceptional patient experience."

- The Web site for Riverside Methodist Hospital contains a patient and visitor guide that aims to provide consumers with information about what it's like to be a patient at the Columbus, OH, hospital, part of the Ohio Health System. The guide provides the patient with information such as "Getting ready for your hospital stay," "What to expect during your stay," and "After you go home." For friends and family, there's information about visiting hours, infection control, the gift shop, and local accommodations. Another section on the site, "Health questions and answers," provides health reference information for a variety of diseases and conditions.

- Responding to quality data published online by the Colorado Hospital Association, Exempla Healthcare, a three-hospital system in Colorado, provides patients with a guide to help them understand commonly used terms and numbers in the reports.

- Paul Levy, CEO of Beth Israel Deaconess Hospital in Boston, started a blog about a year ago called "Running a Hospital." In his blog, Levy tells jokes, talks about current events, and even reports his hospital's performance in key areas such as infection rates and patient satisfaction. Levy has even gone so far as to challenge competing hospitals to publish these data in a similar manner.